Mental Health,
Service User Involvement
and Recovery

First published in 2010
by Jessica Kingsley Publishers
73 Collier Street
London N1 9BE, UK
and
400 Market Street, Suite 400
Philadelphia, PA 19106, USA

www.jkp.com

Library of Congress Cataloging in Publication Data
Mental health, service user involvement and recovery / edited by Jenny Weinstein.
p. cm.
Includes bibliographical references and index.
ISBN 978-1-84310-688-3 (pb : alk. paper) 1. Mental health services--Great Britain--Citizen participation. I. Weinstein, Jenny, 1947-
RA790.7.G7M465 2010
362.196'8900941--dc22
2009018625

British Library Cataloguing in Publication Data
A CIP catalogue record for this book is available from the British Library

ISBN 978 1 84310 688 3
eISBN 978 0 85700 212 9

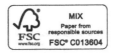

Mental Health, Service User Involvement and Recovery

Edited by Jenny Weinstein

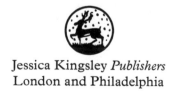

Jessica Kingsley *Publishers*
London and Philadelphia

Acknowledgements

To Dr Philip Kemp, whose vision, dedicated groundwork and steady support made this project possible.

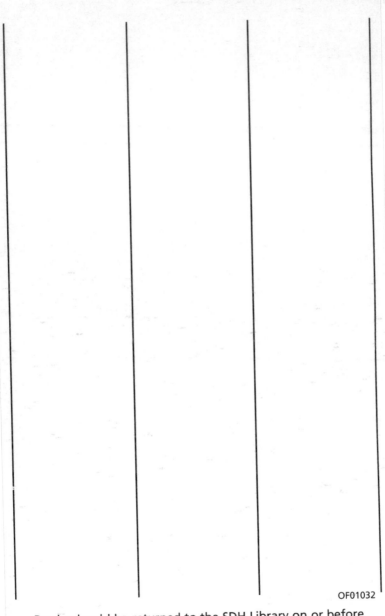

OF01032

Books should be returned to the SDH Library on or before
the date stamped above unless a renewal has been arranged

Salisbury District Hospital Library
Telephone: Salisbury (01722) 336262 extn. 4432 / 33
Out of hours answer machine in operation

Contents

Introduction

Jenny Weinstein

The experts by experience who contributed to this book and their academic colleagues take the view that people with mental health problems can be enabled to Recover if they are empowered to participate fully in decisions about their own treatment and care and if they are spared the stigma and discrimination that have historically exacerbated mental distress. Furthermore, service users must also play a meaningful role in designing, planning, evaluating, researching and commissioning services. In the authors' view mental health workers will be better able to understand and participate in this kind of partnership when service users are fully involved in professional education and training.

Policy guidance in relation to user involvement and more personalized services was initiated in the *National Service Framework for Mental Health* (Department of Health 1999) and has evolved incrementally towards a vision of Recovery (Department of Health 2001), better services for women (Department of Health 2003a), challenging racism and being more culturally competent (Department of Health 2003b), ensuring social inclusion, self-determination and choice for service users (Care Services Improvement Partnership 2006; Department of Health 2006) and transforming the nature of adult services through a programme of personalization (Department of Health 2007). Through the voices and experiences of people who are at different stages in their own Recovery process, the book evaluates the degree to which service users' day-to-day experiences have actually improved in the light of these developments and provides good practice guidance for taking the agenda forward.

The word Recovery is written in this text with an upper case 'R' to denote that its meaning in the context of mental health discourses generally is different from the dictionary definition of the word 'recovery', which usually means a return to a normal healthy state following illness or accident. Recovery, as defined in dictionaries, may be impossible for many people with long-term mental health conditions but there is no reason why they should not be able to live a fulfilling life and participate in normal aspects of communal activities such as work, education, leisure, sport and relationships. As Julie Gosling explains in Chapter 2, Recovery is about taking back control of one's own life and being back in the driving seat. The individual has the power to manage her or his own Recovery (Deegan 1997; Roberts and Wolfson 2004); Recovery is a process of growth and adaptation to an illness or disability not a cure for all symptoms (Perkins and Repper 1996); and the process is unique to each individual (Young and Ensing 1999).

Similarly the word Black is written with an upper case 'B' because the word is not used to denote 'race' but to signify individuals, groups and communities who experience discrimination because of their skin colour.

BACKGROUND AND PROCESS OF PRODUCING THE BOOK

Context

The idea for this book arose from a programme of learning devised, in consultation with users, by one of the book's authors, Dr Philip Kemp, for students of mental health nursing at London South Bank University. The course module was entitled 'User Involvement and the Politics of Mental Health Practice' and its content is pretty much reflected in the chapter headings of this book. Some mental health professionals are keen to involve service users but are not sure how to go about engaging with potential user colleagues. In order to demonstrate that this is easier than it may appear, this introduction will briefly describe how the collaboration with the range of user authors was achieved.

Meeting the user authors

New to Southwark and mental health teaching in 2004, I visited all the local community mental health resources in the area and spoke to service users about my need for assistance. There was considerable interest and enthusiasm and people were invited to put their names down to attend an information meeting at London South Bank University. Approximately 40 people came and the objectives of the teaching and roles that they might play were explained. I also provided details of briefing and support available, the fees that would be paid and the implications in regard to benefits.

From this meeting, approximately 12 service users started to assist regularly with the mental health teaching. Two contributors to this book, Sharon Hamshere and Geoff Worley, joined us via the Lorrimore Drop-in and Ejaeta Egoh came via Simba, a Black user-led resource. Meanwhile the local South London and Maudsley National Health Service (NHS) Foundation Trust had initiated a user-led 'training the trainers' initiative in its education and development department and Aloyse Raptopoulos was introduced to us through this route. Humphrey Greaves was already teaching at a neighbouring university so, hearing about our work on the service user grapevine, he approached us to see if he could be of use. Humphrey and Aloyse have each contributed two illuminating chapters to this book (Chapters 3 to 6). Humphrey put me in touch with his colleagues at the local MIND organization, who co-authored Chapter 9 on service development and planning.

Before coming to the university, I had worked in a large charity called Jewish Care, where part of my job involved finding out what service users thought about services and making recommendations for improvements and developments. Significant changes were made to the way in which this process was managed by involving mental health service users in the design and implementation of quality assurance reviews (Weinstein 2006). One outcome was that 'sheltered' employment projects were replaced by real work or volunteering placements and an education and training department was established for users. I heard of the tremendous work being undertaken by this department after I had left the organization and those involved agreed to write about their work on combating stigma in Chapter 8.

I met Advocacy in Action at a conference in 2005. I was so impressed with their presentation that I kept all their material and contact details carefully. I was delighted when Julie Gosling agreed to share her extensive knowledge and experience to contribute Chapter 2 on Recovery and involvement to this book.

Process of development

A group of academic and service user contributors to this book met at London South Bank University to plan the content and agree the proposal. Our intention was to ensure that in every chapter, the service users' voices and perspectives would be heard directly and each chapter was completed with a conclusion and some guidance for good practice.

We had intended, with the user contributors, to work as a collective in the production of the book – all acting as co-editors. Unfortunately, but understandably, the publisher required one individual to be accountable for the final manuscript. Nevertheless, the content was agreed collaboratively and everyone has been invited to critique other chapters.

Content of the book

Chapters 1 and 2 offer a starting point for the rest of the book in terms of background and philosophy. Chapter 1 by Dr Philip Kemp provides a historical analysis of service user involvement and sets the context by examining the developments within a social and political perspective. Chapter 2 by Julie Gosling lays out a set of values and ethos for involvement and Recovery that was developed by her organization, Advocacy in Action, brought to life with examples from the work of the group.

Chapters 3 to 6 are written by authors who have used services and drawn from their own experiences to illustrate what helps and what hinders a good Recovery. In Chapter 3, Humphrey Greaves, a self-employed user consultant, explains how his personal determination to work and make a contribution enabled him to Recover from severe mental illness, despite the many hurdles and obstacles he found in his path. In Chapter 4, Humphrey reflects on the part played by racism in his original breakdown and how he used his own experience to support other service users from Black and ethnic minority groups. Chapter 5, written by former service user, education and holistic health consultant Aloyse Raptopoulos, offers a challenging first person account of her mental health breakdown and the consequent 'treatment' she received. In reflecting retrospectively on her experience, which she regards as a spiritual initiation, Aloyse pinpoints key issues of bad and good practice. In Chapter 6 Aloyse charts her road to Recovery, highlighting the key turning point when she took control of her own treatment and care.

Chapters 7 to 9 are written in collaboration with service users from different settings. Chapter 7 is written by Jenny Weinstein with support from 15 service users. They discuss the degree to which services have become genuinely person-centred and how far service users feel fully involved in their own care. Chapter 8 considers the impact of stigma on Recovery and suggests ways of challenging discrimination both at a national level – explored through the literature by Jenny Weinstein and in a case example described by a group of Jewish Care service users. In Chapter 9, providing case examples to illustrate the points, Jenny Weinstein and Southwark MIND service users argue that although there are now legal requirements for user involvement in planning and developing services, and many structures to make this happen, some service users still feel that it remains a lip-service or tick-box process and as yet has not had a real impact on service quality.

Chapters 10 to 12 address user involvement in research and in education and training. In Chapter 10, Professor Tony Leiba critically evaluates his experience of working collaboratively with service users in a research project and draws out lessons for good practice. Chapter 11 describes the in-depth work undertaken by Philip Kemp through his project to develop creative methods of involving service users in the classroom and, most importantly, demonstrates the impact of user involvement on students' learning. Chapter 12 presents the innovative work undertaken by Tom Wilks and Liz Green, who involved young care leavers in training social workers. It describes how, through critiquing, developing and delivering training materials, young people had a real impact on social work students as well as improving their own mental well-being and self-esteem.

In Chapter 13 the editor, with a few words by Humphrey Greaves, summarizes the key themes of the book and looks forward to the future for user involvement.

REFERENCES

Care Services Improvement Partnership (2006) *Our Choices in Mental Health: A Framework for Improving Choice for People Who Use Mental Health Services and their Carers.* London: CSIP. Available at www.parliament.uk/deposits/depositedpapers/2009/DEP2009-0074.pdf, accessed on 12 May 2009.

Deegan, P.E. (1997) 'Recovery and empowerment for people with psychiatric disabilities.' *Social Work in Health Care 25,* 3, 11–24.

Department of Health (1999) *National Service Framework for Mental Health.* London: Department of Health.

Department of Health (2001) *The Journey to Recovery: The Government's Vision for Mental Health Care.* London: The Stationery Office.

Department of Health (2003a) *Mainstreaming Gender and Women's Mental Health Implementation Guidance.* London: The Stationery Office.

Department of Health (2003b) *Delivering Race Equality: A Framework for Action.* London: The Stationery Office.

Department of Health (2006) *Our Health, Our Care, Our Say: A New Direction for Community Services,* Cm 6737. London: The Stationery Office.

Department of Health (2007) *Putting People First: A Shared Vision and Commitment to the Transformation of Adult Social Care.* London: Department of Health.

Perkins, R.E. and Repper, J.M. (1996) *Working Alongside People with Long Term Mental Health Problems.* London: Nelson Thornes.

Roberts, G. and Wolfson, P. (2004) 'The rediscovery of Recovery: Open to all.' *Advances in Psychiatric Treatment 10*, 1, 37–48.

Weinstein, J. (2006) 'Involving service users in quality assurance.' *Health Expectations 9*, 2, 99–109.

Young, S.L. and Ensing, D.S. (1999) 'Exploring Recovery from the perspective of people with psychiatric disabilities.' *Psychiatric Rehabilitation Journal 22*, 3, 127–134.

CHAPTER I

Introduction to Mental Health Service User Involvement

Philip Kemp

INTRODUCTION

Few would doubt that user involvement has now established itself as a significant feature in the landscape of mental health service provision. Service users are increasingly involved in a wide range of activities, including policy advice and development, service planning and commissioning, individual care planning, mental health research, service provision, service evaluation, professional education and independent advocacy all of which are discussed in more depth throughout this book. Some might argue that current developments are open to criticism and that there is still some way to go (Campbell 2005; Lakeman, Walsh and McGowan 2007). Nevertheless, it does appear that a critical point has been reached. Many of the areas of development are self-reinforcing and serve to maintain the momentum towards increasing user involvement and a reversal in the direction of travel is hard to conceive. It is important to understand, therefore, that 'user involvement' is no passing fad.

This chapter provides an overview of the development of user involvement in mental health services in the UK. One of the reasons why user involvement should not be considered as a transient phenomenon is that it is embedded in, and in part arises from, fundamental changes within wider society which have taken place in recent decades, in particular changes in the way the state relates to its citizens. This relationship also influences how health and welfare services are structured and in turn how mental health care and support is provided. At the same time social changes have opened up opportunities for sections within society to articulate a 'voice' in a way that was previously circumvented. One such voice arises from people who have experienced mental health difficulties or who have used mental health services. The following range of influences that have contributed to the development of user involvement in mental health services will be considered in turn:

- wider social changes

- citizenship and participation

- government policy and user involvement

- the growth of the 'user movement' in mental health

- professional and service responses to user involvement.

WIDER SOCIAL CHANGES

To fully appreciate why user involvement in mental health services has developed to current levels, it is important to step back and examine how society itself has changed in important ways. These societal changes have served to provide some of the momentum for increasing user involvement in mental health services.

One important social change is that there has been a trend towards more participative forms of governance. It is argued that the problems of modern society have become more complex (for example, health inequalities and social exclusion), and sometimes have acquired a global dimension (for example, climate change, economic fluctuations, decisions of transnational businesses and supra-national organizations). Governments often lack the ability to respond effectively as they do not have full control over situations affecting their citizens (Newman *et al.* 2004). Moreover, traditional forms of representative government through elected bodies appear to be an insufficient means of reconnecting citizens with governing institutions and processes. As a result new forms of governance are evolving:

> in which the state must collaborate with a wide range of actors in networks that cut across the public, private and voluntary sectors, and operate across different levels of decision-making. (Newman *et al.* 2004, p.204)

Both these developments – the efficacy of responding to complex social issues and public disaffection with traditional political processes – have led to developments in alternative forms of governance. In this context Newman (2003) makes a distinction between the role of the state in 'governing' through direct forms of control and a shift towards 'governance' in which the state must collaborate with a wide range of stakeholders at all levels of public policy decision-making. The public participation policies, discussed below, need to be viewed within this wider context.

The dispersal of power from the state, however, does not necessarily equate to a loss of power. Governments have had to develop new forms of control as a response to this process of fragmentation. In UK public policy this has taken the form of framework documents, targets, performance indicators, service standards, customer charters, arm's length regulatory bodies and so on (Newman 2003). Implicit within such developments, however, is the increased reliance on networks across public, private and voluntary sectors with which governments have had to develop collaborative partnerships, and which thus provide an impetus to wider public involvement. Within this dichotomy of central control and dispersal of power, however, potential tension and conflict can arise because of differing underlying motives for public participation as viewed by different sets of participants.

A second significant social change is that we live in a more consumerist society in which members of the public have increased expectations about what they aspire to in life and in terms of standards of service demanded. In the age of the internet and a 24-hour news culture, the public are also generally more knowledgeable and better able to make informed decisions. Such developments serve to reinforce the need to express preferences and also to seek redress if dissatisfied.

This leads to a third area of social change in that these developments impact on how the public view professionals and the relationship between professional workers and people who use services. It has been argued that we live in times where there is a 'crisis of trust' (O'Neil 2002) and this appears to have been particularly associated with politicians in the latter stages of the Blair government. However, within public services the evidence in relation to public trust is contradictory. There is some evidence to support the idea that the public retains trust in health care professionals (British Medical Association 2003). However, policy responses appear to accept that there has been a loss of trust and that this has partly been fuelled by high profile cases where the actions of health and social care professionals have been called into question. Notable instances include the inquiry undertaken by Dr Ian Kennedy into professional practices at Bristol Royal Infirmary (Department of Health 2001), the public and political concern arising from organ removals without parental consent at Alder Hey Hospital (Redfern, Keeling and Powell 2001) and the case of Dr Harold Shipman (Smith 2004). For example, a key recommendation of the inquiry into Bristol Royal Infirmary was increased involvement of patients and the public in health care and this led directly to changes to professional regulation in the NHS Reform and Health Care Professions Act (HM Government 2002):

> We agree that the voices of citizens, patients and their carers should be on the inside, influencing every level of service. (Department of Health 2001, para.31)

In social work the recurrence of similar concerns in relation to the care of children at risk, such as Victoria Climbié (Laming 2003) and Baby Peter (Ofsted 2008), has had a similar effect on policy makers to introduce more robust measures for regulating the professions and how they operate. Nursing has been included in this broad sweep and mental health care has also been beset with a series of high profile public inquires questioning professional competence and attitudes in the series of 'hospital scandals' during the 1970s (Martin 1984) and 'community care' scandals in the 1990s (Reith 1998).

A paradoxical situation has therefore arisen whereby the defining qualities of professionals – autonomy, special expertise, client centredness – are seen as problematic by policy makers and in turn questioned by the public. The policy response has been to introduce initiatives designed to protect the public against the activities of professionals.

CITIZENSHIP AND PARTICIPATION

The concept of citizenship is central to any consideration of individuals' relationship to, and participation in, society. As Dwyer (2002) points out, the ways in which we define citizenship are indicative of the values that underpin how we view society. Conceptualizations of citizenship inform how users of welfare services are perceived by the state, and in turn potentially influence the nature of user involvement. Ideas of citizenship, as they are manifested within UK welfare policies, have evolved in significant ways as the prevailing political orthodoxies of successive governments have changed. The struggle for basic civic and political rights culminated in the acquisition of social rights after World War II with the establishment of the Welfare State. This enshrined the concept of universality, and rights to free health care, education and income maintenance. This social democratic model of the welfare state prevailed in Britain until the 1970s when its sustainability became increasingly called into question in the changing economic environment leading to what became known as the 'crisis in welfare' (Mishra 1984). The election of Ronald Reagan in the USA and Margaret Thatcher in the UK inaugurated a new orthodoxy whereby neo-liberal or 'New Right' philosophies were applied to the role of the state in public policy and welfare provision. This neo-liberal philosophy was characterized by a reduced role for the state, privatization, low taxation, an undermining of public monopolies and the application of market approaches to public policy. The new orthodoxy conceptualized the citizen as a consumer articulating individual (and family) interests within a market economy. This was implicit with the introduction of market principles to the health service and community care reforms following the publication of the White Papers *Working for Patients* (Department of Health 1989a) and *Caring for People* (Department of Health 1989b), which were translated into the National Health Service and Community Care Act 1990 and were intended to 'give people a greater individual say in how they live their lives and the services they need to help them do so' (Department of Health 1989a, para.1.8).

Accompanying the changes in health service and community care during the 1980s and 1990s, therefore, were a range of consultative mechanisms including patient satisfaction surveys, consumer audit, citizens' juries and health panels (Pickard 1998). These were intended to ensure that health service organizations involved the public and gave them a 'greater voice' (NHS Executive 1995).

The reality of how far users of health and community care services were able to exercise consumer choice and influence the market has been much criticized (for example, Paton, Birch and Jordan 1998). This was particularly the case in respect of mental health service users where monopoly provision tended to remain the norm, and where there are particular challenges in facilitating individual mental health service users in the exercise of choice or articulating their needs. There is the additional problem of how far a consumerist model fits with service users who were compulsorily treated under the 1983 and 2007 Mental Health Acts (Barnes and Shardlow 1997; Sayce 2000).

A further factor challenging the relevance of a consumerist view of citizenship in mental health services is the problem of social exclusion. This imposes structural constraints on the 'practice of citizenship' and the ability of many people with mental health difficulties to participate as members of their communities (Office of the Deputy Prime Minister 2004). Thus stigma (Crisp 2005), social inequalities associated with mental illness (Murali and Oyebode 2004); the additional influences of ethnicity (Bhui *et al.* 2003) and gender (Owen and Milburn 2001) all represent structural factors that undermine the notion of citizenship in respect of mental health service users.

With the advent of New Labour in 1997 there was a further re-conceptualization of citizenship. This involved a change in focus of service users from 'consumers' to a new rhetoric of 'active citizens' (Milewa, Valentine and Calnan 1998) and the promotion of the idea that citizens should have direct involvement in decision-making. Under this approach user involvement is presented as a means of empowerment based on social participation. However, a central component of the idea of active or social citizenship is conditionality; the idea that eligibility for social welfare benefits and services is conditional on certain obligations to society. There is an emphasis on individual responsibilities over individual rights. This approach is seen in a number of social policy areas: housing, with measures to tackle tenants who engage in antisocial behaviour; unemployment benefits, whereby claimants are required to demonstrate specific efforts to seek employment, the responsibility of lone parents and people with a disability to accept jobs or training where this is possible; pensions, with the expectation that individuals take on increased responsibility for their financial needs in old age (Powell 2000). Thus citizens need to demonstrate their entitlement to welfare through work, contributing to their own future welfare and by requisite behaviour. Failure to fulfil these obligations could potentially exclude individuals from welfare. This view of social citizenship has some important implications for how users of welfare services are characterized. Social citizenship based on conditionality rather than universal entitlement, it has been argued, runs the risk of promoting exclusion rather than inclusion (Dwyer 2002).

Changes in the way citizenship is conceptualized thus give rise to potential areas of conflict and tension. Participation within a 'consumerist model' is conceived of as a means of eliciting consumer preferences in order that services can be developed and shaped to meet consumer needs more effectively. The emphasis is on consumer rights, information, access, choice and redress, in contrast to a 'democratic model' of participation that values participation itself as an enriching and empowering process for service users. It emphasizes involving service users in decision-making and mobilizing them to participate effectively (Rowe and Shepherd 2002).

However, the *policy driven* consumerist and stakeholder views of citizenship, although accompanied by a participatory rhetoric, appear at odds with democratic views of participation frequently associated with service users and service user groups and organizations. Harrison and Mort (1998) go further and argue that user involvement is a strategy used by policy makers to legitimize the decisions they make: '[user involvement is] technologies of legitimation which can be seen as a means by which managerial legitimacy is maintained in a context of increasingly pluralistic policy area' (Harrison and Mort 1998, p.68).

GOVERNMENT POLICY AND USER INVOLVEMENT

While there might be debate about policy intentions, it is clear that public participation and user involvement has become a central policy imperative informing health and social care services and practices (Hogg 2009). In terms of formal structures, Community Health Councils (CHCs), introduced in 1974, were the principal manifestation of public participation in the health service for nearly 20 years. Since the election of the Labour government in 1997, a range of statutory structures and duties aimed at involving the public in the NHS have been established, and this policy initiative continues to evolve. In the *NHS Plan* (Department of Health 2000) the government signalled a policy focus for the NHS on 'Patient and Public Involvement' (PPI) and the intention to set up new arrangements to promote and facilitate this. This included the abolition of CHCs in 2003 in the face of some opposition (Covey 2000; House of Commons 2003). Section 11 of the Health and Social Care Act 2001 assigned a legal duty on NHS Trusts, Primary Care Trusts and Strategic Health Authorities to establish arrangements for involving the public. With the abolition of CHCs their functions were dispersed among a range of successor organizations. The inspection function and public representation role was taken over by Patient and Public Involvement forums (PPIfs) which were implemented from 2003. Forums were established in each NHS Trust and Primary Care Trust. The statutory powers of PPIfs included the right of access to health care premises; the right to request written information to which NHS Trusts and PCTs had to respond within 20 days; and the right to refer matters to local authority Overview and Scrutiny Committees (OSCs). The intention was that PPIfs would also feed back to NHS Trusts public and patient experiences of health services as a means of stimulating service improvements.

PPIfs were supported by a new national organization, the Commission for Patient and Public Involvement in Health (CPPIH), which became operational from 2003. The complaints function of CHCs was taken on by Patient Advice and Liaison Services (PALS) and the Independent Complaints and Advocacy Service (ICAS). Local authority Overview and Scrutiny Committees provided additional scrutiny of proposals for local organization and service changes within the NHS.

Less than 18 months after becoming operational, the government announced its intention to abolish the CPPIH in July 2004 (although not implemented until April 2008) following the passing of the Local Government and Public Involvement in Health Act (HM Government 2007). In addition PPIfs have been replaced by Local Involvement Networks (LINks). The government's case for replacing PPIfs with LINks (see case study on LINks in Chapter 9) is that they were not representative of their local communities and that they were too bureaucratic. In addition, it was argued that they did not reflect subsequent changes to the NHS such as commissioning and the developments in primary care. Most significantly perhaps their remit did not extend to the social care sector which LINks will now cover (House of Commons 2007).

Other recent developments include the introduction of Foundation Trusts which have a duty to engage with their local community and encourage local people to become members of the organization. They also have to establish a Board of Governors or Members Council whose members are not otherwise involved in the running of the Foundation Trust. The Healthcare Commission (formerly the Commission for Health Improvement – CHI) in its main inspectorate function conducts patient survey programmes and as part of its work programme utilizes service user consultation exercises on specific issues.

Mental health policies and user involvement

References to user participation within mental health policy pronouncements, such as the *National Service Framework for Mental Health* (Department of Health 1999a), the *NHS Plan* (Department of Health 2000) and *Supporting People* (Godfrey *et al.* 2003) initiative similarly adopt the rhetoric of patient and public participation. Within the mental health field service users individually, or as members of user groups and organizations, are involved in a wide range of activities: national policy formulation; local service planning and development; campaigning; advocacy; service provision; service monitoring; user-led research; and professional education and training. At the level of individual care delivery, policy and professional practice prescribes the involvement of service users (Department of Health 1999a, 1999b). Users themselves expect to be involved in making decisions about their own care and treatment. There are increasing requirements for service providers and mental health professionals to develop services that are user-sensitive and based on what users themselves feel are most helpful to them.

However, the rhetoric on increased participation and empowering service users raises a further contradiction within the context of mental health care. This relates to government concerns about risk and dangerousness which many commentators (for example, Peck and Parker 1998) argue has been the main driving force behind mental health policy initiatives since the early 1990s which, it is argued, has tended towards the coercive. This was reflected, for example, in protracted debates about the government's amendments to reform the Mental Health Act 1983 prior to the eventual passing of the Mental Health Act 2007 (see, for example, Scott-Moncrieff 2005). This included the contentious proposal to extend compulsory powers to treat some people with mental health problems living in the community.

THE GROWTH OF THE 'USER MOVEMENT' IN MENTAL HEALTH

In contrast to 'top-down' policy initiatives, any account of user involvement in mental health services must include the longer tradition of 'bottom-up' demands from mental health service users themselves for greater involvement. The organization of collective user activity has been a significant development in the mental health field since the late 1980s (Campbell 2005; Crossley 1999; Rogers and Pilgrim 1991; Wallcraft, Read and Sweeney 2003).

One explanatory framework through which the rise and development of mental health service user organizations can be viewed is in terms of the 'new politics' and 'social movement' theory (Crossley 2002). Social movements represent a new form of politics whereby campaigns about contentious issues within advanced Western societies no longer take the form of traditional institutionalized conflict but are increasingly extra-parliamentary. Moreover, such campaigns, it is argued, are less concerned with problems of economic distribution (the 'old politics') but rather concerned with quality of life, equal rights, individual self-realization, participation and human rights.

Typical of this trend has been the growth of social movement organizations operating within the 'new politics' in such fields as gay rights, the feminist movement, Black power, environmentalism and disability politics. It is argued that the rise of mental health user and survivor organizations is consistent with this trend and that they share many of the characteristics associated with new social movements (Barnes 2002; Crossley 1999; Rogers and Pilgrim 1991).

A key social movement within psychiatry was the 'anti-psychiatry movement' which flourished in the late 1960s and 1970s. Crossley (1998), in his analysis of the anti-psychiatry movement, points out that although it was not a user movement, it did provide an oppositional philosophy which influenced early user organizations. The anti-psychiatry movement was a source of inspiration to many who were instrumental in early user organizations in the 1970s, many of whom went on to become involved in the rapid expansion of user organizations that took place in the late 1980s and 1990s (Campbell 1996). The person most closely associated with the anti-psychiatry movement was the psychiatrist R.D. Laing (although he eschewed the term anti-psychiatry). According to Crossley (1998), there is considerable evidence that Laing found strong support among service user activists. His book *The Divided Self* (Laing 1990), first published in 1960, was widely read. His influence is found in the early user groups in the 1960s and 1970s and served a key function in igniting the development of user organizations. It provided for users an alternative discourse of psychiatry which resonated with their own personal experiences.

Crossley (1999) dates the origins of a user social movement to 1971 with the formation of the Mental Patients Union. It has been observed that levels of social activism cluster and that the late 1960s and early 1970s was a period of high levels of activity across and within a range of social movements. The clustering of activity arises as the opportunities and incentives for other groups to develop become apparent. It must be remembered, therefore, that the conditions which allowed for the emergence of anti-psychiatry were wider than the field of psychiatry itself and are associated with the counter-culture movements of the 1960s and civil liberty debates at that time. Within the mental health field, other groups developed such as the Community Organization for Psychiatric Emergencies (COPE) and the Campaign Against Psychiatric Oppression (CAPO).

The extent of the influence of these early user groups is not clear but Crossley (1999) points out that many service users active at this time went on to contribute to the rapid development of user organizations that arose in the late 1980s and 1990s. The mid-1980s was a turning point in the development of user organizations in the UK. Alongside wider societal trends that gave rise to new social movements, it is often possible to identify 'trigger events' (Crossley 1999). In the case of the mental health user and survivor movement, it appears that the World Federation of Mental Health/MIND Conference held in Brighton in July 1985 was such an event. Guest speakers visiting from the Netherlands, where patient councils had become established, made a strong impression on users who attended (Rogers and Pilgrim 1991). Following this conference the number of service user organizations rapidly grew and they became active in an increasingly wide range of areas. The community care reforms after 1990 provided an additional stimulus and contributed to official acceptance and encouragement of the role of user organizations in contrast to ignoring their relevance as in the earlier radical phase of development during the 1960s and 1970s.

New social movement theory provides an explanation, therefore, of the emergence of different (and critical) voices outside of the institutional context of psychiatry. Within the traditional institutional framework under which psychiatry has operated, mental health service users have been relatively disempowered. New social movement theory suggests that with the development of social movement organizations there is increased symmetry between different participants within psychiatry. Thus the late twentieth and early twenty-first centuries saw the development of a 'communicative space', within which the voice of service users could be heard and included in the dialogue of psychiatry and mental health care and treatment. Ideologically, it provided users with the opportunity to formulate an alternative discourse constituted by their experience and their identities as users in a different form.

PROFESSIONAL AND SERVICE RESPONSES TO USER INVOLVEMENT

Social changes, government policy imperatives and an increasing acceptance of the values underlying user involvement, mean mental health professionals have increasingly incorporated user perspectives in the way care is delivered and how they relate to service users, and user involvement is becoming more widely embedded in mental health services.

Within the culture of mental health service provision, a different value base is emerging based on partnership and collaboration with service users. A number of user-focused philosophies imbued with such a value-base have become increasingly influential. Normalization (Wolfensberger

1972) has been one influential ideological theme, informing community care in particular. The approach promoted the importance of citizenship enabling social participation and personal decision-making for otherwise marginalized people, including the right to decisions concerning life choices. It moved the focus of quality from services to users' lifestyles (Wistow and Barnes 1993).

A policy-driven approach to user-focused care delivery is evident in the *Ten Essential Shared Capabilities* (National Institute for Mental Health in England (NIMHE) 2004). The *Ten Essential Shared Capabilities* are user-focused competencies intended to be generic for all mental health workers and have become an important source of occupational standards for informing service developments, job specifications and professional education and training.

This was followed by the 'recovery approach' being heavily promoted by the Department of Health (National Institute for Mental Health in England 2005; Care Services Improvement Partnership, Royal College of Psychiatrists and Social Care Institute for Excellence 2007). This user-focused philosophy has been defined in the following way:

> Recovery is what people experience themselves as they become empowered to manage their lives in a manner that allows them to achieve a fulfilling, meaningful life and a contributing sense of belonging in their communities. (National Institute for Mental Health in England 2005, p.2)

As argued throughout this book, the application of a Recovery philosophy by mental health professionals and service providers is an important development as it provides for a service-user-informed, values-based approach to mental health care and support. It involves a reappraisal of how services and mental health professionals relate to service users and potentially provides a structure for genuine collaboration.

CONCLUSION

This chapter has examined the sources of increasing momentum towards more participatory health and social care services in terms of social change, public policy, user movements and developments within professional practice. However, there remain some important questions about user involvement in mental health services in terms of its future development. First, in influencing professional practice and the adoption of user-focused philosophies, how to apply them in practice and develop the associated changes of attitude this requires; second, in the target-driven world of public service provision, how to safeguard against tokenistic responses to user involvement by service providers; and third, how to reconcile user involvement with policy and professional pressures to provide a 'safe' mental health service. These are challenging questions but the momentum towards increasing user involvement that is now evident means that such questions should in time produce positive responses.

REFERENCES

Barnes, M. (2002) 'Bringing difference into deliberation? Disabled people, survivors and local governance.' *Policy and Politics 30*, 3, 319–331.

Barnes, M. and Shardlow, P. (1997) 'From passive recipient to active citizen: Participation in mental user groups.' *Journal of Mental Health 6*, 3, 289–300.

Bhui, K., Stansfield, S., Hull, S., Priebe, S., Mole, F. and Feder, G. (2003) 'Ethnic variations in the pathways to and use of specialist services in the UK: Systematic review.' *British Journal of Psychiatry 182*, 105–116.

British Medical Association (2003) 'Public retains great trust in doctors, Mori poll shows.' BMA press release, London 18 February.

Campbell. P. (1996) 'The History of the User Movement in the UK.' In T. Heller, J. Reynolds, R. Gomm, R. Muston and S. Pattison (eds) *Mental Health Matters: A Reader.* London: Macmillan with the Open University.

Campbell, P. (2005) 'From Little Acorns: The Mental Health Service User Movement.' In A. Bell and P. Lindley (eds) *Beyond the Water Towers: The Unfinished Revolution in Mental Health Services 1985–2005.* London: Sainsbury Centre for Mental Health.

Care Services Improvement Partnership, Royal College of Psychiatrists and Social Care Institute for Excellence (SCIE) (2007) *A Common Purpose: Recovery in Future Mental Health Services.* London: SCIE.

Covey, D. (2000) 'Muzzling the watchdog.' Guardian, 13 September. Available at www.guardian.co.uk/society/2000/sep/13/guardiansocietysupplement6, accessed on 12 May 2009.

Crisp, A.H. (ed.) (2005) *Every Family in the Land: Understanding Prejudice and Discrimination Against People with Mental Illness*, revised edn. London: Royal Society of Medicine.

Crossley, N. (1998) 'R.D. Laing and the British anti-psychiatry movement: A socio-historical analysis.' *Social Science and Medicine 47*, 7, 877–889.

Crossley, N. (1999) 'Fish, field, habitus and madness: The first wave mental health users movement in Great Britain.' *British Journal of Sociology 50*, 4, 647–670.

Crossley, N. (2002) *Making Sense of Social Movements.* Buckingham: Open University Press.

Department of Health (1989a) *Working for Patients: The Health Service, Caring for the 1990s*, Cm 555. London: HMSO.

Department of Health (1989b) *Caring for People: Community Care in the Next Decade and Beyond.* London: HMSO.

Department of Health (1999a) *National Service Framework for Mental Health.* London: The Department of Health.

Department of Health (1999b) *Effective Co-ordination in Mental Health Services: A Policy Booklet.* London: The Stationery Office.

Department of Health (2000) *The NHS Plan.* London: Department of Health.

Department of Health (2001) *Learning from Bristol: The Department of Health's Response to the Report of the Public Inquiry into Children's Heart Surgery at the Bristol Royal Infirmary 1984–1995.* London: Department of Health.

Dwyer, P. 2002 'Making sense of social citizenship: Some user views on welfare rights and responsibilities.' *Critical Social Policy 22,* 2, 273–299.

Godfrey, M., Callaghan, G., Johnson, L. and Waddington, E. (2003) *Supporting People: A Guide to User Involvement for Organizations Providing Housing Related Support Services.* London: Office of the Deputy Prime Minister.

Harrison, S. and Mort, M. (1998) 'Which champions, which people? Public and user involvement in health care.' *Social Policy and Administration 32,* 1, 60–70.

HM Government (2002) *National Health Service Reform and Health Care Professions Act.* London: The Stationery Office.

HM Government (2007) *Local Government and Public Involvement in Health Act.* London: The Stationery Office.

Hogg, C. (2009) *Citizens, Consumers, and the NHS.* Basingstoke: Palgrave MacMillan.

House of Commons (2003) *Patient and Public Involvement in the NHS.* Health Committee, Seventh Report of Session 2002–3, London: The Stationery Office.

House of Commons (2007) *Patient and Public Involvement in the NHS.* Health Committee, Third Report of Session 2006–7, London: The Stationery Office.

Laing, R.D. (1990) *The Divided Self.* London: Penguin.

Lakeman, R., Walsh, J. and McGowan, P. (2007) 'Service users, authority, power and protest: A call for renewed activism.' *Mental Health Practice 11,* 4, 12–16.

Laming, H. (2003) *The Victoria Climbié Inquiry,* Cm 5730. London: Department of Health.

Martin, J.P. (1984) *Hospitals in Trouble.* Oxford: Blackwell.

Milewa, T., Valentine, J. and Calnan, M. (1998) 'Managerialism and active citizenship in Britain's reformed health service: Power and community in an era of decentralisation.' *Social Science Medicine 47,* 4, 507–517.

Mishra, R. (1984) *The Welfare State in Crisis.* Brighton: Wheatsheaf.

Murali, V. and Oyebode, F. (2004) 'Poverty, social inequality and mental health.' *Advances in Psychiatric Treatment 10,* 3, 216–224.

National Institute for Mental Health in England (NIMHE) (2004) *The Ten Essential Shared Capabilities for Mental Health Practice: Shared Capabilities for All Mental Health Workers.* London: NIMHE.

National Institute for Mental Health in England (NIMHE) (2005) *NIMHE Guiding Statement on Recovery.* London: NIMHE.

Newman, J. (2003) *Modernising Governance: New Labour, Policy and Society.* London: Sage.

Newman, J., Barnes, M., Sullivan, H. and Knops, A. (2004) 'Public participation and collaborative governance.' *Journal of Social Policy 33*, 2, 203–222.

NHS Executive (1995) *Patient Partnership: Building a Collaborative Strategy.* Leeds: NHS Executive.

Office of the Deputy Prime Minister (ODPM) (2004) *Mental Health and Social Exclusion: Social Exclusion Unit Report.* London: ODPM.

Ofsted (2008) *Joint Area Review Haringey Children's Services Authority Area: Review of Services for Children and Young People with Particular Reference to Safeguarding.* London: Ofsted, Healthcare Commission and Her Majesty's Inspectorate of Constabulary.

O'Neil, O. (2002) *A Question of Trust: BBC Reith Lectures 2002.* Cambridge: Cambridge University Press.

Owen, S. and Milburn, C. (2001) 'Implementing research findings into practice: Improving and developing services for women with serious and enduring mental health problems,' *Journal of Psychiatric and Mental Health Nursing 8*, 3, 221–231.

Paton, C.W.H.K., Birch, K. and Jordan, K. (1998) *Competition and Planning in the NHS: The Consequences of the NHS Reforms,* 2nd edn. Cheltenham: Stanley Thornes.

Peck, E. and Parker, E. (1998) 'Mental health policy in the NHS: Policy and practice 1979–1998.' *Journal of Mental Health 7*, 3, 241–259.

Pickard, S. (1998) 'Citizenship and consumerism in health care.' *Social Policy and Administration 23*, 1, 226–244.

Powell, M.A. (2000) 'New Labour and the third way in the British welfare state: A new and distinctive approach?' *Critical Social Policy 20*, 1, 39–60.

Redfern, M., Keeling, J. and Powell, E. (2001) *The Royal Liverpool Children's Inquiry.* London: House of Commons.

Reith, M. (1998) *Community Care Tragedies: A Practice Guide to Mental Health Inquiries.* Birmingham: Venture Press.

Rogers, A. and Pilgrim, D. (1991) 'Pulling down churches: Accounting for the British mental health users' movement.' *Sociology of Health and Illness 13*, 2, 129–148.

Rowe, R. and Shepherd, M. (2002) 'Public participation in the New NHS: No closer to citizen control?' *Social Policy and Administration 36*, 3, 270–290.

Sayce, L. (2000) *From Psychiatric Patient to Citizen.* London: MacMillan.

Scott-Moncrieff, L. (2005) 'Treatment and care under mental health law.' *Legal Action,* November, 7–9.

Smith J. (2004) *The Shipman Inquiry: Fifth Report – Safeguarding Patients: Lessons from the Past – Proposals for the Future,* Cm 6394, London: House of Commons.

Wallcraft, J., Read, J. and Sweeney, A. (2003) *On Our Own Terms: Users and Survivors of Mental Health Services Working Together for Support and Change.* London: Sainsbury Centre for Mental Health.

Wistow, G. and Barnes, M. (1993) 'User involvement in community care: Origins, purposes and applications.' *Public Administration 71*, 3, 279–299.

Wolfensberger, W. (1972) *The Principles of Normalization in Human Services.* Toronto: National Institute of Mental Retardation.

CHAPTER 2

The Ethos of Involvement as the Route to Recovery

Julie Gosling

INTRODUCTION

I propose to explore involvement and Recovery through my 20 years' experience inside a user-led organization called Advocacy in Action (AIA) as I feel that this is where I have learned most about what works best within partnership. By reflecting on AIA's collective history as experts by experience, I hope to draw out some of the wider principles of involvement and Recovery.

AIA is a network of service-eligible people, founded in 1990 on the principles of human value and potential, mutual support and non-conditional acceptance. Membership has involved people with learning disabilities, physical or sensory disabilities, homeless people, people with existing or previous alcohol or drug habits, older people, carers and people surviving the care system or surviving mental illness. Some of us use services, others resist, and others still have been rejected by services or are invisible to them. Between us, we share a wide range of beliefs, faiths, cultures, ethnicity and experiences that enrich our understanding and mutual support.

Although our professional allies helped us steer our own routes, stood staunchly by our side and used their good power to navigate opportunities for us and are thus part of our history and our success, AIA is not funded by any particular body or organization because we do not want to be tied to anyone that might compromise our values or dictate how we work. We charge for particular projects that we undertake. This includes direct work with individuals or groups as well as teaching, consultancy, research and evaluation. We come to work to make justice, not money, and all workers remain unpaid. However, we charge commercial rates to statutory bodies such as trusts, local authorities or universities and ask little or no fee from service users and carers.

WHAT WE MEAN BY RECOVERY

The most important aspect of our understanding of Recovery is that we own the definition, not the professionals. This means that we decide what we mean by being 'well' – we do not need someone else to tell us whether we are ill or well. Some service users say that they feel well when they are listened to, others when they are able to reject services and cope on their own. My definition is that Recovery is about reclaiming power and control and moving back into the driving seat. I know from my personal experience that it is impossible to *empower* any human being other than oneself. We are not *empowered* from the outside, we have to snatch power back and this is crucial to Recovery. The powerful among us can only look at the power held and use it responsibly, let it go where it can be shared, or pass it on to others.

Understanding a user perspective on Recovery is also about recognizing the achievements of individuals who may lead unsafe lives. Amy Winehouse and Stephen Fry are role models but there are many less well-known people who can live lives and achieve desired goals despite their substance use, untreated mental illness or risky lifestyles that others might find unacceptable. There seems to be pressure from society to protect people from themselves and to try to make them live the same lives as everyone else. I wonder if this is about a deep-rooted fear of 'the other' and a need to control, to sanitize, to medicalize and to cure?

Yet when I reflect on some of the greatest human achievements, they spring from the opposite – from risk and adversities rather than comfort and stability. Many people choose not to be healthy and not to be secure – some choose to deny or to live on the edge of safety or to opt out in a search for something less tangible. Inspiration, faith, political convictions, altruism, 'belonging' – there are diverse ideals that cause individuals and communities to relinquish the so-called benefits of 'civilized society'. Is it less 'mad' to suffer the depression, anxiety and stress that we know is so rife among people pursuing the rat race in order to attain career success, material possessions or society's approval? What can we learn from alternative communities – street drinkers, rough sleepers, travellers and all the other duckers and divers who hack out their own chosen lifestyles, social and moral pathways?

How involved can someone ever be in their own Recovery when they are living a life not of their choosing and in a place where they would prefer not to be? These arguments are relevant for people in hospital on section, people with dementia forced to live in care homes and people receiving treatment against their will. The importance of having control over your own life is illustrated in the case examples (names changed in all examples) described below:

> Don had severe physical disabilities and learning disabilities. His language was limited and he was doubly incontinent. However, he was discharged from a residential establishment to live in an ordinary home with a dedicated carer. The carer was told by the social workers that he and she would benefit if Don attended a day centre every day. Don loved his new home and resisted every day in protest when the transport came to take him to the day centre where he soiled himself every day. One day, the carer decided to follow Don's wishes and support him to stay at home. She was told by the social worker that she would receive no additional funding or support for not complying.
>
> Within four weeks Don became clean and dry. The only power he held was the use of his bladder and bowels to testify to his needs and wants. Once he felt listened to, he stopped advocating for himself in this way.

> An Irish older man named Seamus lived in a damp and dirty house with five other Irishmen who had lived and worked together over years of thankless and gruelling work on the building sites of England and now lived and drank together in squalid and impoverished conditions.
>
> Seamus was in the final stages of life but decided against the clean hospital bed and support of hospice services in favour of remaining with his companions and dying as he had lived. The men enabled home-based services to make his final days comfortable so that Seamus, tended by his companions, planned his own funeral, put his affairs in order and died a peaceful death.

In all my experience I have not come across anyone who was not capable of being involved whatever their illness or disability. For example:

> When Moon Tong first joined our support group he displayed control by banging his head on the wall, smashing his possessions, ripping off his shirt and burning himself with cigarettes. But he came to realize that people cared about him – understood that he was accepted as he was and that his impairments or behaviour were not a problem to us; so, although he did not say anything in the group, he turned up every week, and his self-harm diminished as he found other positive ways of joining in.

User involvement in their individual treatment and care is clearly critical to Recovery but user involvement can also contribute to Recovery in situations where users become part of a team or group like AIA with a sense of purpose. People start to feel depended on and needed and gain a sense of responsibility. Their expertise, experience and knowledge are recognized and they become aware of their potential to grow and gain new skills. Gaining positive feedback from interventions such as teaching or consultancy restores a sense of self-worth. Power and powerlessness begin to shift and the balance changes. Involvement can enable people to feel powerful again and this is part of Recovery.

Our work has become widely known so we are often asked to help 'set up' a self-advocacy group in other parts of the UK or other countries. We always refuse, saying:

> We will not set up enablement or inclusion initiatives for someone else. If we do that it becomes top down and defeats the object. What we will do, however, is work alongside powerless people. If they decide *for themselves* that they wish to organize around the principle of empowerment or involvement, we will support them to do this as long as they need us but they must always be in the driving seat.

In this way, we have assisted groups all over the world to find and achieve their own definition of Recovery.

INVOLVEMENT WITH PROFESSIONALS

I want to begin by differentiating between two types of involvement. First, there is the one that is underpinned by AIA values:

- involvement = collaboration

- involvement = innovation

- involvement = empowerment

- involvement = redistribution.

Second, there is the involvement that has been hijacked by service providers for their own ends where:

- involvement = compliance

- involvement = containment

- involvement = coercion

- involvement = incorporation.

The latter happens where service users are the invited guests at the spectacle but they never decide who to invite. Involvement is often a conditional invitation to join someone else's ball game where rules and goal posts are already set. You can join the team as long as you play ball. We are expected to always be on our best behaviour and not to upset anyone. It relies on the premise that as responsible partners we are all of us good obedient citizens who will learn the inclusion game, stick to the rules and play fair. Naughty citizens don't get to join in.

Professional colleagues upset each other all the time and are expected to know how to 'manage conflict' but if a service user upsets professionals the whole process of user involvement comes into question. Examples from our experience include the following:

- A memo sent to all departments by the chair of a social services committee instructing that they must 'have nothing to do with Advocacy in Action'.

- A day service manager threatened to sue his service users over a video in which they talked about what they liked and disliked about the service.

- A director of a joint Learning Disabilities and Mental Health Service who told me that 'self-advocacy is about speaking your mind without making the manager angry'.

- A local MIND group whose funding was withdrawn soon after it was taken over by service users.

- A secure hospital where we had been called in to help the patient communities organize a speak-out group following the death of a patient who had ingested his own vomit while left strapped to a toilet. 'You won't get me to speak out,' one patient told me, 'it's different here – not like a prison where you know your sentence and you know when you can get out. If you upset them in here, they are just going to slap on more time and you'll end up never getting out again.'

The distress caused to the user is not always taken into account and appropriate support is rarely forthcoming for him or her.

Because of the government policies on user involvement outlined in other chapters of this book (see, for example, Chapters 1, 7 and 9), service providers have had to take on what I call the 'outer wrappings' – that is the language and the processes of involvement; they have to be able to tick the user involvement boxes. However, in practice what they do is top down and designed to incorporate users or neutralize their dissatisfaction. Thus, as illustrated in Chapter 9 on involvement in planning, we are asked our opinion but if it does not suit, it can be ignored; we are invited to join existing boards or committees but no real efforts are made to ensure that we understand the proceedings and are empowered to make a genuine contribution. One of the most upsetting outcomes is where involvement becomes an opportunity for theft or piracy by professional and academic treasure seekers – the colonizers who write clever books about our ideas and then promote themselves as 'experts' in involvement. On some occasions such people have even invited us to come and be trained in 'user involvement' rather than acknowledging us as the experts and the instigators.

While it is vital to be aware of the distinctions between 'good' or 'bad' types of involvement, I have, over time, learnt that a combination of both good and bad elements may come into play, singly or simultaneously within the complex engagements through which we involve ourselves with professional providers and educators so that the course is not a linear one. The notion of a staged journey towards some participatory ideal does not quite capture the turbulence of involvement and the raft of different motivations that may be present in shared activity towards some joint horizon of apparent common outcomes.

While I would always wish to associate myself with the nobler participatory principles, I am not quite as zealous and insistent about this as I may have been earlier on in my work. I have learnt that positive results can and do spring from a variety of motivations and even when underlying principles and practice have less apparent integrity and are more control driven, involvement can and does make a difference in the lives of distressed, disaffected and powerless people, and professionals can be helped to improve their involvement practice.

Nevertheless, there have been rare occasions when we have become involved and regretted it. I remember the shock waves caused when we handed back a substantial fee because we realized that our commissioners' values did not comply with our own and also the fury of an individual university educator with whom we disinvolve because of her shoddy involvement practice. Any decision on our part to disengage is usually redefined by our ex-partners as our incapacity or some inherent flaw within our own practice, but we know different. I cannot begin to describe the relief of off-loading a bad partnership and the ensuing feelings of strength and validation that soon replace any residual guilt. These experiences help us to empathize with professionals who may find themselves in contexts where there is dissonance between their values and those of the agencies where they work and we try to help them devise appropriate strategies for managing this.

INVOLVEMENT WITH SERVICE USERS

Advocacy

Advocacy is a vital component of user involvement and this has now been recognized by government and written into the Mental Health Act 2007 as a requirement. However advocacy, in our experience, is a good example of an involvement process that either can genuinely benefit the service user or can be used by providers for their own ends. For example:

> Two women with a range of disabilities and considerable strengths, Amita and Paulette, had lived successfully within the community with a dedicated carer for many years. Unfortunately, the carer herself became too unwell to continue caring so new placements needed to be identified. The women's involvement in choosing their new homes was non-existent and, despite them being active working members of their local community, they were allocated to nursing home places. When the proposed plans were opposed, the professionals agreed to provide the women with advocates but these advocates were not chosen by the service users. The service users wanted their carer who knew them well to be their advocate. With the carer's support and the involvement of local politicians, the women finally won huge battles with arrogant professionals to have a say in their own lives. One now lives on a coastal farm where she enjoys feeding sheep and sowing crops while the other lives with a new family that she helped to select who enabled her to maintain her chosen lifestyle.

In another example AIA was asked to work with a group of service users of a decommissioned day centre to help counsel them through their loss. We politely declined this role but offered to assist service users to organize themselves to challenge rather than to come to terms with service loss. We must be very careful as advocates that our involvement truly serves the needs, views and aspirations of the individuals and communities we serve and that we are not incorporated by the providers to serve their interests.

Boundaries

One of the main differences between the way AIA works with people and the way professionals work is the issue of boundaries. There are absolutely no 'us' and 'them' boundaries in the way we work with people. Because of the absolute belief we have in one another, the things we do and the way we are with people, I think that involvement for us is more a way of life and a set of values than just a process that applies to bits of our lives at certain times – it is an ethos – it is a set of codes by which we try to live a life that includes and respects everyone.

If professionals wish to participate in one of our initiatives, they have to embrace our values. For example:

> A local medical centre asked us to set up a drop-in and self-advocacy project with some of the patients in their practice. This has been very popular and successful. The doctors sometimes like to pop into the drop-in and they are welcome to do so. However, when they do, it is not in the role of 'Dr Smith', it is as themselves – a person – to be called by their first name and to interact with everyone on equal terms.

A tragic example of how 'boundaries' can prevent people from receiving help when they most need it is related below.

> Peadar had survived many life traumas and disaffections from childhood onwards ending up sleeping rough in a cardboard box, addicted to alcohol and with a diagnosis of bipolar before managing to pull his life together and landing a super job as 'involvement officer' for a Mental Health Trust. He was, of course, a feather in the cap of the Mental Health Trust, whose staff trumpeted their achievements about how involvement had led to Recovery.
>
> Unfortunately a relapse in his mental health provoked another period of instability and a return to alcohol after some years' abstinence, which led to him being beaten up in the city centre one night. This incident set him back and he started to work from home. One day he telephoned colleagues to say that he felt too ill to even get any food in for himself. The response was an email advising him that he could order in food via Tesco online. Some days later he was found dead in his room after police forced entry. It was estimated that he had been dead for four days.
>
> An associate at the Trust regretted that although he was their involvement officer, they had not involved themselves in his life. They maintained the boundaries because he was a 'work colleague'. No

one knew where or how he lived; no one had gone to knock on his door with a bag of groceries or a get well card. Not one of them, in the end, had been there for him.

Responsibilities of involvement

A lesson from this sad story is that involvement brings with it huge responsibilities. Whenever people become involved with AIA, we take them on unconditionally and we accept responsibility, in partnership with them, for all aspects of their lives. We involve ourselves in their lives as well as involving them in our work. This is because the whole person comes with the package – not just the bit of experience we want to make use of – otherwise there is a risk that involvement will be exploitative. We must remember that when we open things up for vulnerable people, we have to shoulder the consequences. A bit of challenge and hope can build people up but there is also the risk that they might then go back down. Involvement means being there when needed. For example:

> I personally have stood with an Irish elder, our backs against the door as the landlord and his hard men tried to illegally evict him. The week before, we stood together in front of a class of students.

Involvement is a two-way street – involvement is not just about us being involved in your lives – it is about you being involved in ours. For example:

> When I was living alongside Leroy, an autistic man, I would hold him and rock with him, thus becoming involved in his world – rather than trying to force him into mine. I found his world to be richer and more fascinating than mine – gentler and more tolerant than so-called civilized society. He was validated and healed by my being involved in his world. I was healed and validated by his acceptance of me.

Risk and 'challenging' behaviour

As mentioned above, I have not met anyone who could not be involved. This includes people with so-called 'challenging behaviour'. In our experience, rather than being angered or frightened by people's behaviour or responding in a controlling or threatening way, it is vital to try to enter their world, to understand the logic – from their perspective – of their adverse reaction or behaviour. When people feel understood, or even just accepted, trust can be built and these trusting relationships assist Recovery. Bruno Bettelheim (1950) suggested that when someone has been very angry or upset or behaved in a challenging way it is helpful to find something positive to feedback to them such as 'you came out of that really well' rather than offering only a negative or critical response. Criticism and negativity will only escalate the person's distress while acceptance can de-escalate heightened emotions. Most challenging behaviour is about survival in the only way possible at that moment in time.

This applies to risk assessment. Professionals in mental health are currently extremely risk conscious and risk averse. It is essential that service users are involved in their own risk assessment. If asked, they know what situations trigger their illness and how these might be managed. They can also make advance directives about how they would like to be dealt with should they become ill or should their behaviour become risky. Service users should be involved in the assessment of risk both to themselves and to other people (Langan and Lindow 2004). Involved does not just mean in a meeting but throughout the whole process of discussing risks, exploring the extent of agreement or disagreement and focusing on what the service user considers important. For example:

> Mary, Nazira and Marie, who had learning disabilities, did their own risk assessment in relation to going to work in a charity shop in the city centre. They assessed the risk of the journey and coping with traffic and crossing busy roads. They assessed the risk of stairs that would need to be negotiated by one of them, who had a physical disability. They assessed the risk of being treated 'like children' by people in the shop, who would not show them the proper respect. But most important, they assessed their own strengths and how these would enable them to overcome the risks.

Involving service users, especially in matters that concern risk, can sometimes cause conflicts with carers who have different perspectives and needs. Some over-protective or concerned carers feel extremely sceptical about their loved ones with mental health problems or learning disabilities being involved in decisions about their own care. Carers can put significant pressure on professionals in this respect and service users can be squeezed into a corner.

In our experience it is vital to recognize that both service users and carers have unmet needs but these are different. By being in conflict with each other, they both lose out. We try to help service users and carers to campaign to have their own specific needs met – fighting their own battles – side by side – but in the same war.

DIFFERENT WAYS OF BEING INVOLVED

The demand for user involvement has been bottom up, as outlined in Chapter 1, but the government now deems involvement a good thing and is requiring involvement through top-down policy requirements referenced in many parts of this book. So it is now possible for service users to be involved in the following ways:

- to witness and be witnessed in all that is done for us and on our behalf

- to be involved in our own care

- to be involved in planning, delivering or evaluating services

- to be involved in strategy

- to be involved in campaigning, resistance, subversion and challenge

- to be involved in education and research

- to be involved in innovation and new alternatives

- to be involved in capacity building.

There is no hierarchical process here – users can be involved in all or any of the above at any one time – depending where they are in their own lives. We dip in and out of involvement depending on energy levels. It is not a static process – we experience 'hot spots' of involvement based on our full understanding of the right to be or not to be involved. Non-involvement is not a step backward or a failure – it is just where we need to be from time to time, and non-involvement may be less about apathy – more about action.

Planning services – your services or ours?

When I consider involvement in service provision, a scenario flashes to my mind: 'service plans → service user views → service decisions → improved outcomes for users'. There always seems to be a given that the service is necessary or unnecessary in the first place and there are no alternatives or choices offered in relation to this major decision – only supplementary, minor embellishments. At AIA we quickly learned along the way that speaking your mind was OK, was rewarded even, when you were involved in mini-decisions such as what colour the walls of the day room should be painted. But when people spoke out against the service itself and demanded alternative types of solutions, the advocacy facility was curtailed; it was no longer necessary or desirable for people to be involved. Advocacy, empowerment, involvement are apparently OK as long as they are toothless! The system appears to be unable to deal with threats; it draws in and ingests what it finds palatable and spits out everything else. The outcome is a diluted compromise that disappoints and disempowers those service users who believed they were being involved and consulted.

At AIA we never agree to be involved in planning services unless we know that the service concerned is needed and wanted by the local community it seeks to serve. For example:

> We were asked by service providers to set up a conference for a group of learning disabled people to encourage them to advocate on their own behalf. We declined to take on this task but agreed that if the group was interested, we would talk with them about the value of such events, and, if they wished, assist them to set up *their own* event along the lines that they considered to be helpful to them.

I do not believe that you can ever be truly healthy or Recover from the conditions that tie you down if you are in receipt of services that make no sense or have no resonance with your individual needs or lifestyle. When we are asked to comment on service development, we are therefore particularly concerned to ensure that the specific needs of all ethnic and culturally diverse groups and people with a range of physical and sensory impairments will be catered for within the proposed service.

I am realistic enough to understand that many of our aspirations about the degree of involvement and decision-making we would want for service users may be unrealistic in the immediate future. Nevertheless we can expect honesty as a baseline about where involvement in service planning begins and ends. Service users need to know from the outset exactly what their involvement will mean and it should not be clouded by frilly wrappings of meaningless words and processes of involvement that contain very little within them. Involvement requires recognition and ownership of the many agendas it serves and openness about whose agendas are the most overriding. If this honesty is present, involvement can produce good results even when coming from less democratic principles and practices – when serving compliance agendas for powerful groups for instance, involvement can still be empowering.

Evaluation

Evaluation and quality assurance are popular buzz words and essential boxes that providers now have to tick. Involving service users provides additional brownie points and this can be really meaningful or it can be tokenistic.

One of the important lessons we learnt was to ensure that the qualities or standards being evaluated were relevant for the users as well as the providers. For example:

> When undertaking an evaluation which involved us following a pre-set standards questionnaire, one of the questions was about whether staff were dressed in a 'neat and tidy' way. A service user evaluator protested, 'It's them lot that's neat and tidy and dressed posh that always puts me down – I'm not judging no one on that!' We realized that we needed to ask our own questions based on issues that service users deemed to be important.

Over the years AIA has refined this into a community involvement process where we visit and revisit community ideas and ideals of what makes good support, what services are required and what 'well-being' means to different people. Examples of questions that we think are important are:

- How safe does it feel to live here and how satisfied am I with the level of safety?

- Is this a place where I can say 'yes' and 'no' and be confident that my views will be considered?

- Do I know what this service costs and where the funding is coming from and managed?

- Am I satisfied with the level and quality of the provision?

Involvement in education and training

AIA has written about involvement in education elsewhere (Advocacy in Action *et al.* 2006) and see also Chapters 11 and 12 in this book on the subject, but I would like to summarize a few points here from the service user perspective. For service users, being involved in education and training can mean that our anger, pride and power are all validated. This is not about therapy or Recovery for us but we do gain satisfaction from investing in a better generation of care workers. It is essential that our involvement is not tokenistic or managed in a patronizing way as this is exactly the modelling that would not help students to learn. We need to co-own all the structures and processes and not just be brought in as a tick box exercise. When this is done properly, it is rewarding to see the results of our intervention immediately. The structured critical reflections of students enable presenters to hear about the positive changes that learners intend to make. We ourselves develop and learn from the interactions which help to increase compassion and tolerance for other people as well as enabling us to gain confidence and skills.

In our teaching, some of our members share their life stories with students to help them gain real insight into what helps and what hinders Recovery and the negative impact that poor care giving can have. This approach has been challenged for being 'voyeuristic' and our response is that 'we engage others in open, honest interactions that demand personal and professional change, described by one student as 'face-to face, nowhere-to-hide connection' (AIA 2007, p.57).

CONCLUSION

When done poorly, involvement can raise expectations and make dummies out of people. Service users must beware of colonization – being gulled into feeling valued when their involvement is really only about meeting other people's agendas. Users must be strong enough to resist poor involvement – practice which sets people up to fail, moves the goal post and is much more about professionals' advancement than ours even when they try to tell us that 'involvement is so good for you'.

We have to ensure that involvement is done well. As service users we refuse to stay out of sight or change to please others – we are not the cause of the problem but its effects – we celebrate both our resilience and our human fragility with pride. Involvement is innovative; expertise and innovation are well demonstrated within the self-help and service user movements. Involvement can heal professionals as well; if the care relationship is sick, involvement is the cure; it leads to empowerment and this can bring improved mutual understanding and tolerance and thence real change.

At AIA we see user involvement as a brilliant survival strategy – turning our problems into a marketable commodity, redefining ourselves and thus shifting the power balance to a more equitable one between ourselves and service providers that reduces isolation and validates the experience of both users and professionals. When undertaken well, the process of involvement builds capacity for all partners – learners, service users, providers and educators – we all develop through learning with and from one another. We believe that in the long term this can lead to political, cultural and societal change for the better.

GOOD PRACTICE GUIDANCE FOR EFFECTIVE INVOLVEMENT

Our many years of experience working with service users, carers and service providers suggests that the following are critical to successful working together:

- involvement on a jointly established platform of values and shared beliefs

- involvement where everyone's power is honestly stated

- involvement where we do not talk about equality only equity

- involvement that can challenge

- involvement on our own terms and for our own benefit and for those we represent

- involvement without retaliation

- choice to opt in and out or to 'dis-involve'.

REFERENCES

Advocacy in Action (2007) 'Why Bother? The Truth about Service User Involvement.' In M. Lymbery and K. Postle (eds) *Social Work: A Companion to Learning*. London: Sage.

Advocacy in Action with staff and students from Nottingham University (2006) 'Making it our own ball game: Learning and assessment in social work education.' *Social Work Education 25*, 4, 332–346.

Bettleheim, B. (1950) *Love Is Not Enough: The Treatment of Emotionally Disturbed Children*. Glencoe, IL: Free Press.

Langan, J. and Lindow, V. (2004) *Living with Risk: Mental Health User Involvement in Risk Assessment and Management*. York: The Policy Press in association with Joseph Rowntree Foundation.

CHAPTER 3

Building a Compelling Future

Humphrey Greaves

I once jeered at the broken man. He slipped away leaving his Yoke for me to carry. It was weigh, weigh too heavy!

(Humphrey Greaves 2008)

A MENTAL HEALTH BREAKDOWN

That's the way this chapter in my life began. In trying to cheer up a work colleague who was going through a difficult time. I laughed at an old tramp making some silly joke… I had little knowledge of mental ill health in those days. How it began? Who it affected? I had vaguely heard of depression but I did not know it was a mental illness.

The year was 1981; I was in my early twenties, a mature student studying for a law degree at the Middlesex Polytechnic. I had done reasonably well in the first assignments; things were looking promising. I was in my first year studying subjects like contract law, the English legal system, the law of tort, and sociology. I worked reasonably hard and I was enjoying life.

I fell out with a friend whom I had recently met at polytechnic and for some reason this had a devastating effect on me. I had some difficulty in making and keeping friends before I went to polytechnic. I guess you could say I was a bit of a loner. I just never seemed to fit in. Maybe it was one rejection too many. I was not particularly close to this friend, so the friend was not to blame. My troubles came prepacked.

I began wandering round the corridors of Middlesex Polytechnic like a lost sheep trying to attend tutorials and lectures, hearing voices of people who were not in the room. Everything seemed spaced out, and I found it difficult to concentrate.

I have never taken illegal substances so there was no obvious cause of these strange experiences. I just thought I had been overdoing it a little.

So I decided to take it easy for a while. I still continued to attend lectures and tutorials, trying not to fall behind in my studies. It felt like everyone was laughing at me, I felt vulnerable and insignificant. I remember, during a tutorial on tort, a lecturer asking me a question about special damage. Special damage is damage that a person or persons suffer that is particular to them such as loss of wages, etc. I knew the answer to the lecturer's question but I just sat there shaking, and shaking. Even then, I had no idea I was ill!

> The Ghost tiptoed back into the tortured Soul; it will haunt the broken man tonight.

It was the morning or the afternoon or maybe it was the evening, surely it was not night time? I was unclear as to what time of day it was. I knew it was the day after my mother's birthday or thereabouts because I remember I had recently given her a birthday present. The year was 1981.

I attempted suicide.

My thoughts were fuzzy and I felt I had fallen down a deep chasm – the deep chasm of depression. I could hear banging on the wall, I knew not from whence it came. I took a knife to slash my wrists. I could not see the point of living any more. As far as I recall I was interrupted by my landlord and rushed to Accident and Emergency. To this day I do not know to which hospital I was taken. I never went looking for the past. It just haunts me.

I returned to my parents' home where I made further attempts on my life but something kept me safe. I could not go through with it. Finally, I put a knife through my chest. All the time the voices in my head were laughing.

I was admitted to a hospital called Claybury. It was a difficult time. The ward I was on had what I called a 'submarine' door, since it rather resembled the doors I saw in the submarine movies. They were heavy doors that had, if I recall correctly, at least two locks to them. These doors would be locked at night. Thank God we never had fire as there were also bars on the windows.

Later I was told I suffered from schizophrenia. This label did not really explain to me the hallucinations, voices and suicidal thoughts that I had experienced. But then nothing ever has. I was given tablets called Pimozide that seemed to help a little.

I thought I would be in hospital for ever; why did they not just let me die in peace? Sometimes on a bad day I still have those thoughts. It took me about six months with the help of tablets and therapy to recover sufficiently to be discharged. In those days the only user involvement I saw was rows and rows of old people in the corridors of the hospital picking up cigarette butts; they looked as though they had been there for ever. 'Is this it?' I wondered.

I did return to the polytechnic but I had to start the first year all over again. It was too much for me; the voices followed me everywhere. The libraries were never silent because the voices were keeping such a racket in my head. I tried to sit examinations but I just could not concentrate. I had failed my degree in law. I was out.

WIDE EYED AND JOBLESS, PRESUMED MAD

Now I was unemployed as well as being mad. As far as I recall, if you had a mental rather than a physical health problem, they did not call you 'disabled' in those days. They called you 'cuckoo', 'barking mad', a 'looney', or said 'he's got a screw loose'. On top of that I am black. How was I ever going to get a job?

My social worker from Claybury Hospital had visited me once or twice but nobody told me about sickness benefit so I signed on. I was unemployed, with a million whispers from the voices in my head as I waited to receive my unemployment benefit.

I felt so ashamed. What happened to my dream of becoming a solicitor or lecturer? I meditated on my grandmother's words: 'You are going to be a big shot!' She had used those words when I was on a visit to the West Indies prior to commencing my law degree studies when I told her I was working in a solicitor's office. She has long since passed away; if she could see me now? I hung my head low and scuttled away. I was on my own.

That is not to say that my parents and sisters did not give me plenty of love and kindness, for which I shall be always grateful. But on one level, when you are unwell, it feels as though you are on your own no matter who is with you. Sadly a lot of people have nobody. I was so blessed I had my parents and sisters and somewhere to live. Nevertheless, mental ill health can be a very solitary experience.

I eventually got a job as a clerical assistant with the Department of Trade and Industry (DTI) after a year of looking for work. Even though I was always battling my demons, I was to stay with the DTI for 11 years, gaining one promotion.

In 1991 my health let me down again and I was admitted to the Campbell Centre, which is part of Milton Keynes Hospital. I had 'lost' my mind again (like you can 'misplace' it?) and I was hearing voices. Sometimes I was so confused that I would get lost when trying to get from one place to another. It was not very comforting since I believed people were trying to kill me. To make matters worse, my thoughts seemed to be escaping from my head. This is not a very nice experience because it is as though you have no private thoughts or secrets. I was diagnosed with paranoid schizophrenia.

STARTING A LONG ROCKY ROAD TO RECOVERY

This, however, was to be a major turning point because while I was in Milton Keynes Hospital I was taught relaxation techniques. Everyone in the ward had to do it. I was amazed at the time that a man who had suffered a recent heart attack also had to do relaxation. We did relaxation once a day, led by either an occupational therapist or a psychiatric nurse. To me the use of relaxation techniques is a good example of empowering service users to be involved with their own care. Learning about stress and about how to relax was perhaps the most valuable skill I have ever developed. I now use relaxation when I am stressed and I have since taught it to other service users in the community. It gives us some control over our lives.

One of the important things I did to keep well after I had been discharged from hospital was to find myself some counselling. I believe the counselling was based on Rational Emotive Therapy, although my memory is hazy now. However, I am still benefiting from the impact. It seemed to open up my eyes to not looking at the past and what has gone wrong but building on the here and now. From the few sessions I had I put together an affirmation which I still use to this very day: 'I have grown in strength from the past and I look forward to the future with great optimism.'

Then on my own initiative I started using a technique called 'Focusing'. 'Focusing' involved getting myself into a relaxed state and then answering specific questions and replying in the 'felt sense' – what was I feeling? – *not* what was I thinking? This helped me to get in touch with how I was really feeling about important aspects or issues in my life. Well, this technique was phenomenal. The next morning as I was casually walking to work, this half-raging voice screamed: 'You never give me any emotional support!' And that's all it said. I immediately recognized that this was the root of my problems. I was always looking for support from others, never from myself. Was it a voice from my psychotic past or a voice from my subconscious, who knows? Who cares? All I know is it gave the direction in which to seek some answers to my mental illness.

While I was on leave from Milton Keynes Hospital I dropped by my workplace in London to ask for my job back. They agreed. I did this on my own initiative! Not a bead of sweat was spilt. I had used the relaxation techniques to keep me calm and focused. I kept my job with the DTI until I decided to leave in 1995. Things had to change because the job I was doing with the DTI was not me. So I parted on good terms and joined the National Schizophrenia Fellowship (NSF), now known as Rethink, having previously gained some experience in a voluntary capacity. I had become restless, and the job as project worker helped me to expand my horizons. I liked interacting with people, I think the modern expression is: I am a 'people person'.

SERVICE USER EMPLOYEE

My job at the NSF would be to run drop-ins in different parts of Milton Keynes. The drop-ins were based in various community halls and a youth club in the town centre. The service users were some fabulous people. They all knew I was a user of mental health services and to some extent this gave us a special bond. They knew I had experienced some of what they were going through and this helped them to believe that there was light at the end of tunnel. You know, no matter how ill they were, they would always ask if I was all right. They were some of the most courageous and caring people I have ever met.

One of the things I set up with my manager was a counselling service accessible in the twice weekly drop-ins. This was well used and service users gained a great deal of benefit from it. You would be surprised at how hard service users are prepared to work at staying well, when they are offered the appropriate support.

In 1998 I left the NSF following my marriage, the year before, to my partner, who was living in London. I was sad to leave, but those who used the drop-ins made such a fuss of my wife and me. They even formed a guard of honour and gave us such lovely presents. I will always treasure my memories of my time at the drop-ins. Amazing!

INTERRUPTION TO RECOVERY – IT IS RARELY A STRAIGHTFORWARD JOURNEY

I married my wife in 1997 when I was 39 years old. We met in London. At last I had met someone who wanted to take a chance on me. I was so happy. We loved each other so much. I will always treasure that feeling. My wife Teresa had three children; the youngest was still at primary school. I knew Teresa had taken a big risk in having me as her husband and I was determined to make a success of our marriage. I told Teresa no matter how ill I got, she must always put her children first so I do not blame her for leaving even though I still moan. In 1998 my depression took a turn for the worse, ultimately causing my marriage to end.

Thus, within a short time of returning to London in 1998 I was back in hospital with depression and by 1999 the depression had got so bad that I was struggling to keep working. In the past I had used Person-Centred Counselling and more lately I was given Cognitive Behavioural Therapy (CBT) by a clinical psychologist. CBT was to prove crucial in my bid for Recovery since my clinical psychologist, as well as helping me face my demons, also put notes on file about what I was feeling and experiencing when I was ill. But I shall save the significance of that until later. The other assistance I was given while remaining in work in the community was that I was allowed respite care from time to time which really helped.

I feel my clinical psychologist's letter to my consultant psychiatrist, which was based on the notes from our sessions, really speeded up Recovery since it gave *context* to my medical symptoms. I believe this helped the doctor to find the right medication quickly because he had a whole picture of me – not just a list of symptoms. In my view, so much time and pain could be saved if practitioners would just listen to the patient first. Whenever there is a conference on mental health that has service users as delegates, the most important thing they say will help all service users is if practitioners took time to listen to the service user.

WORKING AND RECOVERY – NOT JUST GLASS COLLECTING!

At the time of writing, there is a focus on returning people on Incapacity Benefit (IB) to work (Department of Work and Pensions (DWP) 2007). Apparently, IB costs £77 billion each year and 40 per cent of this is paid to support people with mental ill health (Meacher 2008; Perkins 2008). While my own story shows how important being able to work is for Recovery, I do not think that the government's current policy is the best way to support people. In my experience service users want to play a part in their community and continue to make a contribution to the economy. I remember being part of a National Schizophrenia Fellowship lobby of Parliament in 1996 which attracted service users from all over the country to fill up the Grand Committee Room to talk to Members of Parliament. Someone said they wanted a job and someone else from the audience said 'and not just glass collecting!'

It makes me so angry when I hear politicians saying that people were put on IB in order to hide rising unemployment figures. Such sound bites completely miss the point about the way in which people's lives have been ruined; their confidence destroyed; and their families decimated through being called 'mentally ill'. If we are not mentally unwell why did they give us these labels? We are maimed for life. Who will want to employ us once we have a mental health label?

So I was not best pleased when the government minister Peter Hain said that,

> Currently there are many people sitting at home in the belief they are unemployable with no life choices or long term prosperity because they do not think their illness or medical conditions can be catered for in the work place. But this is not the case – many people with such conditions are perfectly able to take successful careers, if the right support was in place. (Daily Mail 2007)

But I was sacked because they could not afford to keep me on by financially supporting me while I was sick. If the government wants people with mental health problems to work, they must make provisions for them to cease work temporarily when they relapse and enable employers to finance this.

My experience of returning to work while being a service user is that it is a gradual process and best attempted when the service user feels well enough. From 2000 when I was hospitalized for severe depression it took me seven years to get a part-time job. And I class myself as being one of the better ones: I was not as ill as some. So what are service users supposed to do? The trouble with glass collecting is that it does not pay the bills.

However, there is supposed to be support and encouragement for people with a disability wishing to return to work but I found, when I approached the Job Centre's disability employment adviser, he was never there and there was no accountability. Employment Support Allowance is replacing Incapacity Benefit (DWP 2008) and I hope when this is implemented, that they make staff accountable for genuinely empowering people to return to work – not frightening them or pressurizing them, which will only make them ill again.

I feel we service users need to ensure the right support is available by getting involved in employment issues that relate to mental health. Another step forward would be to reduce stress in the workplace which can be a trigger for mental ill health in some individuals. We need to ask what the government has done to support and educate employers. Employers are often frightened of people with mental health issues and fear that they may cost more than they will contribute. There is no point in penalizing service users for not getting a job if employers are not helped and encouraged to employ us. On the contrary, I suggest that the government has had the opposite effect by triggering moral panics about mental illness and portraying people with mental health issues in a bad light over so many years.

FINDING THE RIGHT KIND OF WORK

For myself, I spent two years wondering how I would get a job once I recovered. For a long time there was no way I was well enough but I kept on hoping that one day I would get a job and play my part within the family. A medical report that stated I was unlikely to work again just got me mad – that was the last straw. No one was going to tell me I was not going to work again! If no one was going to employ me, I would employ myself. So I did. I tried one or two things like Kleeneze but I was not comfortable with that so I decided to practise as a Neuro-Linguistic Programming (NLP) practitioner. I had already qualified so that is how I started my coaching practice in 2002. I went on to increase my skills by qualifying as a Life Coach in 2004. This just goes to show that if practitioners are prepared to help service users develop their strengths, there are no barriers to their progress.

The key to my being successfully self-employed was that those working with me focused on what *I wanted to do* not what *they thought* I should do. In coaching we call this 'following the client's interest'. The manager of Opportunities, a support organization, and my employment adviser were particularly good at this. I was always coming up with ideas and I was never once told: 'Go away. Do not waste my time'. They would always listen.

In the early days when I first came to Opportunities, within a short space of time I found myself at the manager's door, which was willingly opened to me. Instantly I relayed my desire to set up the Building a Compelling Future Group, a personal development group to help my fellow service users who had had an experience of mental ill health. I offered to do a demonstration for all the staff at Opportunities to see for themselves whether it worked or not. When I approached the manager with this idea, I was recovering from mental illness and unemployed but he said 'I'll arrange for my staff to be here on...'

The demonstration went well; I chose to do an exercise on motivation and a relaxation exercise. The participants seemed to gain significant benefits from it. I was then able to set up the group which was based on NLP and later, Life Coaching. We advertised the Building a Compelling Future course in the local community health teams and encouraged service users to self-refer, although they were all vetted by the Opportunities staff.

I did a series of six sessions per course, each of one hour duration. I had some very determined service users who worked very hard, dealing with some difficult issues. They supported and helped each other. There were some fantastic outcomes – some getting jobs, others going on to further education or moving on in their personal lives. I am so privileged to have worked with them. It was an honour.

As usual the dreaded word 'finance' got in the way and Opportunities was disbanded. But the film group survived and is still running to this day (more about that later). Other groups that were run by service users were the Men's Group, Empowering Women, the Art Group and the New Horizons social group. Each of these groups helped to transform service users' lives and I was told that other health professionals found that they needed to have less input into their clients' care while Opportunities was helping them.

As I mentioned, one of the groups that was established within Opportunities was called 'Inspirational Film Works'. This enabled service users to learn how to use camera equipment, etc. We made short films such as *Portraits of Recovery*, which was shown at the Tate Gallery. We also made a film which was commissioned by Oxleas NHS Foundation Trust called *Community Care Programme Approach*. Inspirational Film Works continues to make cutting edge films despite the closure of Opportunities for financial reasons.

> They take you over and then dump you when they feel it is too costly to continue – leaving you naked and cold.

I was very unhappy about the closure of Opportunities as were my fellow service users. I think we lost something that was beginning to make a real difference. Albert Einstein (1879–1955) is quoted as saying that madness is doing the same thing over and over and expecting a different result. What I do not understand is why, when new ideas work, do we so often as a society, dismiss them and revert back to our old ways? Treating people with mental health problems by using a medical model has been around for hundreds of years yet, even though we know it has serious limitations, we still let it continue in the old way. Nevertheless the Opportunities method of working actually worked successfully in tandem with psychiatry not against it. The financial world seems to have no concept of care – the abacus rules. I blame the money men. Do not mind me, I am only the service user.

Talking back, doing it for ourselves – something inside so strong!

Service users, who were not known for their assertiveness, felt empowered enough to stand up for what they wanted and campaigned to keep my support group going. I am so proud of them! I know it took a lot of guts to do that and they did so without any prompting from me. In fact all the things they achieved were down to their hard work and their willingness to try new things. I simply introduced them to the tools. They had begun to see for themselves that they are part of the solution not the problem. I do not just mean in regards to the campaign but in relation to their own issues.

Again this was achieved through the service users supporting each other. It is so important to encourage service users to support themselves. I have not got a cure for mental ill health and the medical profession does what it can. But the essential part of the equation is the service user. The greatest gift one can give to the service user is optimism and that is magnified if the service user can take part in finding the solution. I wonder if anyone has bothered to collect statistics about the number of times fellow service users have supported each other or in some cases saved the life of a fellow service user. There is little publicity or acknowledgement about the service users that work for mental health charities or as mental health nurses. Little is said about the contribution we make. The emphasis always seems to be on the costs of keeping 'layabouts' on benefit without recognizing our value and worth.

AN ESTABLISHED SERVICE USER TRAINER AND PROJECT WORKER

In my own journey, one of the things that put a sparkle in my eye was a laser beam of hope when I was approached by a senior lecturer at the University of Greenwich to help facilitate tutorials for mental health nursing students giving the service user perspective. My input as a service user and survivor seemed to unravel a whole new world for them that they had not seen before. In addition, I am a freelance consultant coach and I have mentored student nurses in practice.

I work in a similar way with London South Bank University. The work is extremely interesting and I help to problem solve, from a service user perspective, some of the issues nurses have to grapple with. My relationship with the students has helped me to appreciate that nurses are also human and I endeavour to show them that a service user is more than a diagnosis. As a freelance consultant with the London South Bank University, I have been involved in recruiting and selecting students for the mental health programme and I was invited to write this chapter.

I find working with the universities very exciting because it helps me to feel part of the solution. It enables me and other service users to have our voices heard and increases student nurses' awareness of the service user experience. One day these students will be fully fledged nurses and I hope that we will have influenced the quality of the care they give. I guess one could say we are patients and service users who talk back – and because we are not in their care, we talk from a position of strength (see Chapter 11).

That is why I was so elated to come across an organization called Southwark MIND where I am presently employed on a part-time basis as a Black and Minority Ethnic (BME) user development worker (see Chapter 4). Southwark MIND is a mental health charity where everyone involved with it is a service user: it is entirely user run and has been so for approximately ten years to date. Southwark MIND has a User Executive Committee and a User Council, plus all its operational staff are service users. It is mainly a campaigning organization that has fought for service improvements like single sex wards and improved emergency services (see Chapter 9).

I remember, when I used to be a project worker for the NSF in 1995, my manager at the time and I were so proud that we had managed to set up a drop-in run entirely by users. Now I realize that it was just these kinds of early initiatives and the growth of the service user movement that they supported which led to the establishment of fully user-run mental health charities such as Southwark MIND. I think it is absolutely amazing!

MENTAL ILLNESS AIN'T CHOOSE Y

Chasing Shadows and the silent sound
hearing voices there is no one around
my homes just west of the lost and found
cardboard boxes or middle class dwelling
or a stately home there is just no telling
my mind's all gone
so depressed, I'm low, low
high, high let the dices roll
Mental illness ain't choose y!
Don't pass me by because I cry
Don't pass by 'cause you label my mind
Don't pass me by I committed no crime
Just give me your hand in love!

(Humphrey Greaves 2008)

CONCLUSION

People who have endured mental ill health through the centuries have been executed, imprisoned, demonized, held in asylums, ridiculed, taken from their families, sacked from their employment, evicted from their homes, attached to electrodes, forced to have sections cut from their brain, and pumped full of medication. If we are to improve our treatment, we services users need to be involved in service provision, monitoring of health care provision and measuring the quality of the aforesaid.

I personally have spent the past 27 years either trying to get a job or hold down a job with the spectre of mental ill health hanging over me. I have lost some very good friends, have lost some very good opportunities for jobs and lost some very good girlfriends, including losing my wife and family.

Often when one is suffering from mental ill health, family and friends go out the window. Many of us are alone and isolated, so if we are able to make a good friend it is a blessing, not only to the individual service users, but also to society, the economy, etc. 'How come' you say, 'all they do in these day centres and drop-ins is sit around and talk?' I would respond by explaining that if you thought about it, you would realize that if service users return to work they have got to be able to relate to others, if they return to college or school they have got to relate. If they go to the corner shop or just about anywhere they have got to be able to relate. Very often their mental health problems are coupled with the fact that they cannot relate to others because of hearing voices, or because they have become withdrawn because they are depressed. So to my mind closing down places where services users can meet is a false economy.

GOOD PRACTICE GUIDANCE FOR PRACTITIONERS, PROVIDERS AND EMPLOYERS

My advice is that *practitioners* should always *listen to service users* and thus help them to:

- recognize their own strengths and talents

- believe in themselves and never give up

- remain optimistic

- be involved in their own care

- find their own individualized roads to Recovery

- access talking and other alternative therapies.

Service *providers* should always *listen to service users* and thus help them to:

- participate in planning and developing services

- take a leading role in delivering services

- benefit from the strength they can gain from supporting each other.

Having a sense of purpose or, ideally, *getting back to work* is important to Recovery but *employers* must understand that:

- users need support and time to return to employment

- users need support and understanding while they are working

- users may relapse and need time out to recover

- employers need training and support in mental health awareness.

REFERENCES

Daily Mail (2007) 'Why we are such a sick note society.' *Mail Online*, 21 November. Available at www.dailymail.co.uk/debate/columnists/article-495476/Why-sick -note-society.html, accessed on 12 May 2009.

Department of Work and Pensions (DWP) (2007) *Welfare Reform Act 2007*. London: The Stationery Office.

Department of Work and Pensions (DWP) (2008) *Your Guide to Employment and Support Allowance*. London: DWP. Available at www.dwp.gov.uk/esa, accessed on 12 May 2009.

Meacher, M. (2008) *The Reform of Incapacity Benefit: A Response to the DWP Green Paper – A New deal for Welfare: Empowering People to Work*. Available at http:// cep.lse.ac.uk/textonly/research/mentalhealth/MollyMeacher_reform-of-inca-pacity-benefit.pdf, accessed on 12 May 2009.

Perkins, R. (2008) 'Abolish the "Separates" now.' *Openmind 145*, 14.

CHAPTER 4

Circle of One
Experiences and Observations of a BME Service User and Consultant

Humphrey Greaves

> *I sat in my dark and dingy bed sit, depressed and close to tears feeling ashamed.*
> *My job had gone, our house had gone, my wife and my step children had gone,*
> *I was on my own. I was a Circle of One.*
>
> (Humphrey Greaves 2008)

INTRODUCTION

There are times when one reaches a crossroads in one's life and one asks oneself the question – could I have done things differently? I have plenty of those instances in my life. So these writings are not designed to pass judgement but to touch on a few areas highlighting where the 'if only' factor might reside. I do not apologize if what I am about to write seems obvious or simple because health professionals constantly ask the same question: 'How can we get more service user involvement?' It seems that governments and health professionals do not do simple. There are so many complex bureaucratic forms and guidelines when, in a nutshell, they just need to treat service users like human beings – end of story. Too simple? OK, let me take you on a journey.

In my quiet moments I look back and I ask how did that happen? How did I end up being a mental health patient? How did I end up losing my family and so on? As I sit combing my mental health files, thinking of the past and what might have been, I come to multiple conclusions as to why I became mentally ill. One contributory factor, which I do not often share with others, is that there was an issue of race.

The circle of one represents many service users in the community who are, one way or another, not included in society. The government says it is keen on 'social inclusion' (National Social Inclusion Programme 2009) but is it going about it the right way? The circle of one is like an elastic band which always comes back to its original shape. I would say that race issues did affect my mental health and I have seen them affect many of my fellow Black and Minority Ethnic (BME) service users. Although the government has now acknowledged there is a problem (Department of Health 2003), I am not sure that its strategies on *Delivering Race Equality* (Department of Health 2004) are going to be enough to really make a difference.

MY MENTAL HEALTH BACKGROUND

I am a Black African Caribbean whose parents are from Barbados. I was diagnosed in 1981 with schizophrenia at a time when the medical profession seemed to have little understanding of our culture and doctors made little effort to explain why they were doing the things they did. Littlewood and Lipsedge (1989) and Fernando (1995) explain the historical development of Western psychiatry and the evolution of ethnocentric Western psychiatric approaches that failed to meet the needs of individuals from different cultures. Sewell (2009) argues that many barriers remain to be overcome before outcomes for BME service users start to improve. This bears out my own experience. I found there was still this automatic assumption that health professionals could apply their own medical model as if they were in a laboratory – clean and clinical. For some reason they refused to accept that they were dealing with a human being whose illness was closely interrelated to his life experience. There have been improvements in recent years but there is still a long way to go.

Racism is an issue I will come to later, but first I want to talk about cultural issues. In any culture it would seem reasonable to expect psychiatrists to get to know their patient first, even if they just had a brief chat. But in my experience psychiatrists often made recommendations about a person before even meeting them. This 'getting to know you' process is even more important if professionals are working with someone from a different culture. They need more time both to understand the cultural issues that might pertain and also to build trust with the person who may feel particularly frightened and insecure. Sewell (2009) argues that consciously or unconsciously, it is likely that the race of a non-white person being referred will negatively impact on the professional receiving the referral. As Ferns (2005) points out:

> Black service users are particularly prone to being subject to the quick fix of physical or drug treatments where practitioners may feel 'out of their depth' with the complexities of trans-cultural work. Practitioners may not understand behaviour in its cultural and spiritual context and lack an effective theoretical framework to analyse what is really going on. (p.137)

It is also important to know the person as part of his or her family and community. This was the strength of old-style general practitioners (GPs) as they used to practise in Britain and may be still doing in the rural areas. More recently many NHS staff can seem a bit faceless but they expect, because they have the title doctor or nurse, that people will immediately open up to them without any prior relationship building. I suggest that in relation to mental illness this is less likely, particularly if service users are from the Black community (see Coll 2002; Cooper et al. 2006; Sainsbury Centre for Mental Health 2002) who all emphasize the key role that relationships play in building trust and facilitating more effective interventions. Other studies come to similar conclusions. Secker and Harding (2002) interviewed African and African Caribbean service users and found that their experiences revolved around a sense of loss of control and racism underpinned by a feeling that relationships with staff were unhelpful, while African or Caribbean service users from East London (Sandhu 2008) reported that being understood and being listened to would significantly improve their experience of mental health services.

If I am going to have someone treat me medically, I want to know if I can trust them. They may be the most qualified and most capable psychiatrist in the world but if I cannot trust them, there will be no or minimal cooperation from me. I think this lack of trust causes many of the perceived 'challenging behaviour' from mentally ill members of the Black community who do not trust the medical profession. This was exemplified in the case of David 'Rocky' Bennett, a Black service user who died while being restrained in hospital (Norfolk, Suffolk and Cambridgeshire Strategic Health Authority 2003). The head of the government's Delivering Race Equality Project, Melba Wilson, acknowledges that historically, the problems have been about 'fear of the services...not feeling they are understood or their needs are being met' (O'Hara 2008).

When someone from the medical profession refuses to explain things and just sits in silence, as some of my psychiatrists did in the early 1980s and 1990s, I felt disempowered and wondered why I had bothered to keep my appointment. Thankfully they were not all like that. But it was difficult if the psychiatrist refused to answer my questions or build any kind of relationship with me. Sometimes I would be seen by a psychiatrist for less than five minutes. In this brief time, without talking or listening to me, they believed they could provide the correct diagnosis. I might as well have gone to a person who reads Tarot cards.

I found it especially difficult to be heard when I voiced concerns about the safety of my family when I was ill in the late 1990s. I was eventually hospitalized in 2000. I do not remember anyone acknowledging their plight nor did they signpost us to other agencies. Nobody acknowledged that the possibilities of family break up or being flung worlds apart could have an effect on my severe depression. I am sure they cared, but did not know how to deal with it. Nevertheless they should have recognized this as a significant factor in my illness. If only someone from the medical profession had heard me and shown me they understood! Who knows, it might have reduced the severity of my illness or shortened the length of it. They seem to think we are just a bag of chemicals devoid of emotions and feelings. All I wanted was for someone to listen.

The important words are empathic relationship and trust. The professionals are often seen as the enemy rather than the one to be trusted, largely because they make so many decisions about our lives which we have no control over. They can have a significant influence even on our very liberty. Would you tell your story to someone you could not trust? Failure to listen, failure to take into consideration one's culture or ethnicity can damage the service user's health.

MY EARLY LIFE

Changing tack a little, I want to reflect on some of the issues that brought me to the mental health services. I seldom deal with this issue; I guess I normally suppress it but I shall take you to one of the darker regions of my circle of one. This year I found a word that depicts one of the drivers behind my mental ill health; the word is abandonment. To me it is more powerful than discrimination or racism. At least with racism it indicates you are part of something, a group or a race. With abandonment you are completely on your own.

My parents brought me up the best way they could, doing a great job, and I will always be indebted to them, but I experienced abandonment from my late primary school days. No, it is not physical abandonment I am talking about. I am talking about what I experienced as the emotional abandonment by society.

Let me set the scene in the late 1960s and early 1970s when I became aware of this feeling. I was doing what other boys do – I was average, nothing special. While I was at school I became aware of the constant beating of war drums going on in society at the time: it was the war between the races – white and black. Now I never experienced any personal racism while I was at school; perhaps I was lucky. My fellow pupils always treated me with respect and dignity and I am proud to have known them. It was the adults who caused the problems; we kids got along just fine.

I had a particular beef with Enoch Powell, the Conservative Member of Parliament. I would be eating breakfast and Enoch Powell would come on the radio saying Blacks should be sent back to their countries of origin. So in my mind the people of England did not want us. My mum would say that Barbados (the birth place of my parents) did not have enough room for us because they had not catered for us. By 'us' she meant children born in the UK from parents who came from Barbados. So where were we supposed to go? I used to joke with my sisters who were born in England that we would end up bobbing about in a dinghy somewhere between England and Barbados in the middle of the Atlantic Ocean. It is not such a joke these days when one thinks of the Vietnamese boat people or refugees from Somalia or Ethiopia dying on perilous sea journeys to seek new lives. The thing was I never knew when Enoch Powell had finished speaking on the radio or television, whether I would have any friends at all by the time I got to school.

These feelings followed me through school to my brief stay at the polytechnic (see Chapter 3) and on into work, my social life and relationships. I still live in fear of abandonment. Sometimes I just do not seem to belong anywhere. Other British-born Black service users experienced personal racism on the estates where they grew up, in their schools where they were called names or in situations where teachers' expectations were that they were fit only for manual jobs; and then when they entered the job market they were turned down in favour of less qualified white applicants. I am pretty sure these feelings had a major part to play in mine and others' mental health. In any given situation I expect to be rejected and this directly impacts on my self-esteem.

When children are young they do not have the same filters for understanding and analysing information as mature adults. They are not likely to realize that Enoch Powell was a wayward politician. Besides, did other politicians feel the same and just not speak out so clearly? All

I can say is that if one is faced with a bully or a mugger there is no use saying there are plenty of other nice people out there. No! One has to deal with the bully or the mugger in front of you. That is how children deal with the danger; children do not care for society's theories or well-meaning smiles, they confront what is before them. I believe the lack of security and race hatred that was stirred up by some politicians; some media; and the influential right wing anti-immigration parties like the National Front that flourished during the 1960s and 1970s may have damaged many Black Britons who, as a result, were destined to become angry, alienated or mentally ill.

INCIDENCE OF MENTAL ILLNESS AMONG BME COMMUNITIES AND POSSIBLE CAUSES

Professor Fred Hickling, a prominent Caribbean psychiatrist (Francis 2006, p.4), states that 'Most Black psychiatrists in the Caribbean would agree there is a slight increase in Schizophrenia in Black Britons, as you would find in any migrant population', but the statistics paint a more serious picture. The Health Care Commission, Mental Health Act Commission and NIMHE/CSIP (2005) found that mental hospital admission rates were three times the average for Black men and double for Black women. A diagnosis of schizophrenia is nine times more common in Black African Caribbeans, six times more likely in Black Africans and two and a half times more common in non-British whites.

Dr Agrey Burke offers an explanation for this, saying that psychiatrists pigeonhole Black people as 'difficult and therefore in need of restraint, not healing' (Goodchild 2003) so that a Black person is seven times more likely to be sent to a secure unit than a white person. Other theories (Fawcett and Karban 2005, p.46) blame the lack of cultural competence among British mental health professionals who misread signs and, for example, read loud voices as 'aggression' and spirituality as 'madness' or suggest that Black people are more likely to suffer poverty, unemployment and racism which may adversely affect their mental health – the 'Increased Stressors' explanation.

A combination of these causes is illustrated in an interview with a BME service user by the name of Niabingi reproduced on the Healthtalkonline (2006) website in the section Mental Health in Minority Ethnic Communities: Experiences of Service Users and Carers. While she was staying at a BME hostel Niabingi realized that racism had played a major part in her developing schizophrenia:

Well for me that was, that was a positive experience because I hadn't, because I think they thought, one of the diagnosis apart from anything else that had happened you know, in my life and my background they said a lot, that some, some, that my, so you know, what contributed significantly to my mental ill health, and I will use ill health rather than, or mental distress because that would be very good case, was, was, racism. And you, you know you know, that I, looking back I think that was quite an accurate diagnosis. (Healthtalkonline 2006)

The racism came from Niabingi's life experience not the medical profession, but for many years it had not been acknowledged even though it was probably a major contributor to her schizophrenia and needed to be taken into account. Understanding this enabled Niabingi to work towards Recovery. One may say, no one thought to ask her before. I would reply that one cannot be expected to ask all the right questions all the time. What one can do is to listen and follow the service user's interest. To put it simply, listen to the service user's story. I think psychiatrists need to listen to the whole picture be it to do with housing, employment, racism, culture, education, or whatever. Science tends to want to isolate some offending gene, or germ when in reality everything in life is interconnected making it impossible to extract one specific cause. We need to work with service users on all their life issues rather than marginalize them or ignore them.

As evidenced in a study by the Social Care Institute for Excellence (Greene, Pugh and Roberts 2008), it is useful to be aware that BME service users often do not seek help early because of their lack of trust in services so that by the time they encounter the NHS they are more likely to have reached a crisis and therefore to be compulsory detained under a section of the Mental Health Act 1989. It is recommended that far more effort is put into outreach work with BME communities to turn this situation around.

WORKING EFFECTIVELY ACROSS CULTURES

Many communities by the very nature of their culture take time to build relationships. I understand that the Japanese businessman will not do business until he has socialized by having dinner with you first. I am not for a moment suggesting that service users be wined and dined (now there's a thought), but I am highlighting the importance of building a therapeutic relationship that empowers service users to get involved with their own care. For it is my opinion that well-being rests in the service user being part of the solution.

As Black men and women we demand respect wherever we go; the Rastafarians will often greet each other by saying the word *Respect*. I sometimes wonder how many clues the medical profession need. If medical professionals do not show respect to their patients, why should they be shocked when service users do not want to engage with them or to be involved on a larger scale? Gaining the respect of the service user is vital and one of the ways of gaining the respect of someone is to give them respect.

One cannot in my opinion build a therapeutic relationship without acknowledging and taking into account the service user's cultural background. Lewis (2005) states that 'cultural issues play a critical role in the formation and expression of personality. In addition, they are a major determinant in contributing to the conditions in which mental illness arises'. It is therefore really helpful if professionals can make a connection across the cultures. He gives the following example:

> When it comes to empathic understanding, there is established data that indicate that communication flows better when common references to shared realities exist. About a year ago I mentioned to one of my service users from Jamaica that I actually knew who Sizzla was. From that point on, our relationship made a U turn. He started to trust me. It was really significant to improving what we were able to accomplish in the ongoing management of his mental health problem. (Lewis 2005)

Diversity training is useful but to gain a real understanding, one must do more than just attend a training course; courses are an aid not a solution. It is unrealistic to expect one person to understand all the different cultures and it is important that training about different cultures does not encourage stereotyping or making assumptions; everyone from a particular culture will not necessarily have the same life experiences, communication style, spiritual or religious beliefs, dietary requirements, family structures or lifestyle expectations. It is therefore better that professionals ask each individual service user about these and other aspects of their lives so that users can feel more confident about being recognized, understood and able to get involved with their own care.

In the words of Joanna Bennett, sister of David 'Rocky' Bennett (Lyall 2006), 'Cultural awareness won't have any effect on power relationships', so any training provided must help staff reflect on their own relationships with users and the way in which institutions provide services.

MY WORK WITH BLACK AND ETHNIC MINORITY GROUPS

In my life there was always a constant gnashing of teeth, 'You have got to do this by a certain time; you must be in fashion; you have got to be good at sport; you have got to succeed in education' and on and on. There never seemed to be any respite; the television and the radio were always pumping out one command or another: 'You must, do, be, have...' When I was first ill with schizophrenia in 1981, I would hear voices and the radio and the television would persecute me, saying that I was a failure and a misfit. On top of that psychiatrists were starting sentences with 'You'll never...' and I felt I did not belong anywhere.

I have purposely shown the power of words, albeit in their negativity, by references to Enoch Powell but if those words seem negative, think of the power of positive words and encouragement. I have been sharing positive words of encouragement with people wherever I go, regardless of their colour, for many years now. I like nothing more than to bump into someone from one of my personal development groups and watch their faces light up as they excitedly tell me what they have achieved and their plans for the future. And I have also watched service users help each other. Now that is one of the seven wonders of world. As I understand it, people become care professionals because they want to make a difference. Do you remember that feeling when you made a difference? Well, I have news for you – everybody wants to make a difference, especially service users. If you empower them to make a difference, you would have made a difference increasing each other's confidence. Then you will see service user involvement in action.

I carry the scars of psychological pain that no one can see, but I am able to use that pain to try to help other service users whether they are Black or white or from any other ethnic group. I will do my best to help – I guess I am a people person. I am also an upstart, who prefers the quiet revolution to aid evolution if that is possible. I have found service users have similar issues whether white or BME. As aptly put by one service user 'We are all human'. From my experience BME service users are not 'hard to reach' – the explanation often given for not involving them. As an aside I would like to highlight how celebrities with mental health issues, such as Trisha Goddard who hosts a talk show on television, can help to change understanding about mental illness. Tricia's show deals with people's emotional issues on Channel 5; Tricia herself is Black and has suffered from mental ill health. If opportunities are offered in the right way, BME service users will participate very enthusiastically.

Some service users become mental health nurses, some become support workers, and so on. Others like to get involved in the politics of service provision by sitting on committees like the Mental Health Partnership Board (See Chapter 9). I myself am a BME user development worker with Southwark MIND. Southwark MIND run a drop-in called the Cuckoo Club, which is for people who have experienced mental ill health and where all races sit side by side and enjoy each others' company. When I see what has been created by the people of Southwark MIND who are all service users, I step back in wonderment: wow, especially when I think of all the negative press we service users get. They should look at the good things service users do too!

When Southwark MIND identified that there was not enough support for BME service users, it successfully applied for three years' funding from the National Lottery to set up a BME project with three staff members who are also service users – one female BME user development worker, myself as the male user development worker and an administrator. Kindred Minds initially started life being called the 'BME project' but was renamed as a result of a democratic vote at our official launch in 2007. Kindred Minds works so well because both staff and BME services users get alongside each other to make the project work. As well as sharing support and mutually agreed activities, members also help to challenge service provision.

I facilitate a Men's Group and we talk about various men's issues, which range from mental health community issues to personal experiences in a fully confidential setting. Kindred Minds runs a fathers' group for service users, which includes any men who may be thinking of becoming a father and want to look at how mental health may impact on them. As a BME project worker, I also visit acute wards in the Maudsley Hospital, give short talks to the patients and facilitate discussions. Other groups include the Kindred Minds pop-in which meets fortnightly to talk, read poetry, or hear about complementary health and our most recent group – Football Coaching.

Although what I have described does not appear earth shattering, I suggest that it may feel earth shattering for the Kindred Minds members. When you sit in front of a psychiatrist, who often will set the agenda, pace and length of your consultation, having time and space to say what you think and feel to people who listen and empathize is very empowering, especially if you are with others from a similar background with common experiences. An example of helping people to feel more confident and positive is a little exercise I do at the end of a Men's Group called The

Hope Circle. This is where we go around the room each saying what we hope for. Just by changing the emphasis from focusing on problems to thinking about what we hope for helps to lift their mood.

Kindred Minds is also involved in challenging mental health provision by trying to assert the BME perspective regarding services in Southwark. One of the ways we do this is by participating in the Cultural Competency Awareness Group meetings at the Maudsley Hospital. This provides an opportunity for BME service users to work effectively together, giving their views and suggestions with regard to service provision in Southwark. It is Kindred Minds' job to try to facilitate this effectively.

I have had my say in this chapter but I have a lot to be thankful for. Thank you for family and friends; I would not be here without you. Thank you to the psychiatrists, doctors and nurses, etc. But a special thank you to all my fellow service users who I have met along the journey.

Circle of one
I'm a circle of one
you say I'm not the man I used to be
maybe it is because I'm the man I've never been
circles make wheels
wheels carry the wagons and the lorries
that bring the food to the hungry
Maybe my circle of one is one of those missing wheels?
Where would we be without circles?
Without wheels?

(Humphrey Greaves 2008)

Think for a moment…how many people get to say that. The power of the circle. This circle is now closed for viewing. Close the door when you leave.

CONCLUSION AND GOOD PRACTICE GUIDANCE

- Black people remain over-represented in the compulsory end of mental health services and under-represented as receivers of preventive and support services.

- Some Black people remain suspicious and distrustful of mental health services because of previous experiences or what they have heard from people in their community.

- Media images and personal experiences of racism and discrimination impact on the mental health of people within the BME community.

- For the reasons outlined above, Black people often do not report early problems of mental illness and are less likely to benefit from essential early intervention.

- Learn as much as you can about different cultures but do not make any assumptions about service users in relation to their background, religion or culture. Make time to find out about each individual in a respectful and sensitive way.

- Be aware that Black service users may have been affected in some way by racism or discrimination. Make it possible for them to tell you about this and demonstrate your empathy.

- BME service users are not hard to reach if approached in the right way but they may feel distrustful about mental health professionals and services. It is up to you to prove that they can trust you.

- It is sometimes easier for BME service users to participate in projects that are run by and for BME service users where they will feel safe and secure. From this base, they may feel more confident about subsequently participating in other services or groups.

- Like all mental health service users, BME service users have significant strengths and the ability to take control of their own Recovery, if they are enabled to do so.

- Like all service users, BME service users make excellent contributions to supporting each other, providing leadership and facilitation and using the creative arts to aid Recovery.

- BME service users must be involved and consulted in the planning, development and delivery of services.

REFERENCES

Coll, X. (2002) 'Please Don't Let Me Be Misunderstood: Importance of Acknowledging Racial and Cultural Differences.' In K. Bhui (ed.) *Racism and Mental Health: Prejudice and Suffering.* London: Jessica Kingsley Publishers.

Cooper, L., Beach, M., Johnson, R. and Inui, T. (2006) 'Delving below the surface: Understanding how race and ethnicity influence relationships in health care.' *Journal of General Internal Medicine 21*, S21–S27.

Department of Health (2003) *Inside Outside: Improving Mental Health Services for Black and Ethnic Minority Communities in England.* London: National Institute for Mental Health in England.

Department of Health (2004) *Delivering Race Equality in Mental Health Care: An Action Plan for Reform Inside and Outside Services and the Government's Response to the Independent Inquiry into the Death of David Bennett.* London: Department of Health.

Fawcett, B. and Karban, K. (2005) *Contemporary Mental Health: Theory, Policy and Practice.* London: Routledge.

Fernando, S. (1995) *Mental Health in a Multi-Ethnic Society.* London: Routledge.

Ferns, P. (2005) 'Finding a Way Forward: A Black Perspective.' In J. Tew (ed.) *Social Perspectives in Mental Health.* London: Jessica Kingsley Publishers.

Francis, P. (2006) 'UK Blacks at no greater risk of Schizophrenia.' *Daily Gleaner* 6 May, 5.

Goodchild, S. (2003) 'Blacks failed by our "racist" system of care for the mentally ill.' *Independent on Sunday,* 28 September. Available at www.independent.co.uk/life-style/health-and-wellbeing/health-news/blacks-failed-by-our-racist-system-of-care-for-mentally-ill-581480.html, accessed on 12 May 2009.

Greene, R., Pugh, R. and Roberts, D. (2008) *Black and Minority Ethnic Parents with Mental Health Problems and their Children.* SCIE Research Briefing 29. London: Social Care Institute for Excellence. Available at www.scie.org.uk/publications/briefings/briefing29, accessed on 12 May 2009.

Health Care Commission, Mental Health Act Commission and National Institute for Mental Health in England/Care Services Improvement Partnership (2005) *National Census of Inpatients in Mental Health Hospitals and Facilities in England and Wales.* London: Health Care Commission. Available at www.cqc.org.uk/_db/_documents/04021746.pdf, accessed on 12 May 2009.

Healthtalkonline (2006) *'Interview with Niabingi' Mental Health in Minority Ethnic Communities – Experiences of Users and Carers.* Witney: DIPEx. Available at www.healthtalkonline.org/mental_health/mentalhealthserviceusers/Topic/3404/Interview/1779/Clip/11889, accessed on 12 May 2009.

Lewis, P (2005) 'Assessing the Impact of Change on Practitioners.' Presentation at Turning Point – National Black and Ethnic Minority Mental Health Network Conference, Solihull, 3–4 October.

Littlewood, R. and Lipsedge, M. (1989) *Aliens and Alienists: Ethnic Minorities and Psychiatry,* 2nd edn. London: Unwin Hyman.

Lyall, J. (2006) 'The struggle for "cultural competence".' *Guardian,* 12 April. Available at www.guardian.co.uk/money/2006/apr/12/publicfinances.politics6, accessed on 12 May 2009.

National Social Inclusion Programme (2009) *Outcomes Framework for Mental Health Services.* London: National Institute for Mental Health in

England. Available at www.socialinclusion.org.uk/publications/Broadened_Social_Inclusion_Outcomes_Framework.pdf, accessed on 12 May 2009.

Norfolk, Suffolk and Cambridgeshire Strategic Health Authority (2003) *Independent Inquiry into the Death of David Bennett.* Norfolk, Suffolk and Cambridgeshire Strategic Health Authority. Available at www.irr.org.uk/pdf/bennett_inquiry.pdf, accessed on 12 May 2009.

O'Hara (2008) 'In place of fear.' *Guardian,* 5 November. Available at www.guardian.co.uk/society/2008/nov/05/melba-wilson-mental-health-issues, accessed on 12 May 2009.

Sainsbury Centre for Mental Health (2002) *Breaking the Circle of Fear: A Review of the Relationship between Mental Health Services and Afro-Caribbean Communities.* London: Sainsbury Centre for Mental Health.

Sandhu, S. (2008) 'Alternative pathways for Black and Ethnic Minority groups.' *Mental Health Today,* May, 23–25.

Secker, J. and Harding, C. (2002) 'African and African Caribbean users' perceptions of in-patient services.' *Journal of Psychiatric and Mental Health Nursing 9,* 2, 161–167.

Sewell, H. (2009) *Working with Ethnicity, Race and Culture in Mental Health.* London: Jessica Kingsley Publishers.

CHAPTER 5

Becoming an Expert by Experience

Aloyse Raptopoulos

Reality is the greatest brainwashing technique ever successfully utilized and maintained... To control people's action, you need to control their thoughts.

(Sen 2006, p.95)

INTRODUCTION

On 6 December 2001 I was walking down the road in Gypsy Hill (south east London) when I stopped in front of a Victorian house, looked at the numbers of the front door, abandoned all my clothes in the car park and started wandering through the streets stark naked.

A tired sun was going down on the hills. The streets were blaring with rush hour's roars and groans, the air thick with its fumes. I was walking naked among the traffic, oblivious to the cars, waiting for the inevitable to happen. If it meant being run over, so be it. 'What is the point in trying to escape if today is the day I'm supposed to die?' I was ready.

At first I thought taking my clothes off had made me invisible because no one tried to talk to me or stop me. I had shaved my head the day before so maybe people were just assuming that I was pulling a stunt as part of a freak show for some reality TV. South east Londoners are not easy to impress. Only from time to time, I could hear a little child bursting with innocent jubilation: 'Look Mummy, the lady has no hair and no clothes on!' But the mother would pull the child's arm firmly without giving me a look. 'Stop making up stories or you won't get ice cream.'

I was utterly frightened yet felt I had no choice but to keep walking in the freezing cold. At some point I crossed a busy road and a car almost hit me. 'Watch where you're going, you fucking whore!' shouted the rude and distracted driver. I raised my eyes to the sky thinking the end was near, and begged: 'God, if you exist, please make my death less painful than life sometimes is.' At this very moment a man gently grabbed my arm.

> 'Where are you going... like that?' he asked.
> 'I'm walking towards the light.'
> 'Aren't you cold?'
> 'I am, but I can't stop. Let me go...'

I noticed a group of passers-by who were giggling hysterically across the road and became tearful. 'Why don't you wait here for a few minutes?' the man said, dialling a number on his mobile phone.

> 'No, please, don't call the police! I'm going to be punished if I try to escape...'
> 'It's not the police you need, young lady, it's an ambulance.'

Soon an ambulance arrived and two paramedics came out of it. One of them threw a blanket over my shoulders and took me inside. 'What happened?' he asked kindly while his colleague was not even trying to repress a mocking smile. I tried to answer but no sound came out of my mouth. 'Well, that's it!' I thought. 'I'm dead – brain dead.'

The paramedics drove me to a place I did not recognize as a hospital at first. I have no recollection of the journey, or how we ended up in front of a locked door surrounded by a thick window. They rang the door bell; a voice spurted out of the interphone but it took a while before someone came to let us in.

We entered a big shady room where a few people were watching incredibly loud TV; most of them were merely staring at the wall. The paramedics disappeared and a woman who did not introduce herself asked me to follow her. She led me into a reeking room fitted with a broken brown cupboard and two small iron beds. 'This is your room,' she said abruptly. On the floor litter and cigarette butts were everywhere. The blue walls were stained with dirt and had no pictures on them, the windows opaque. I turned around to ask her where I was and what I was doing here but words again refused to cooperate. She had already left anyway.

Later on someone else came to let me know that dinner was ready in the main room. But food was not on the agenda for me, now dressed with a white sheet like Mahatma Gandhi and strongly determined to remain on a hunger strike. Nobody asked me why I would not eat or if I needed clothes but it was the least of my worries. I was far more preoccupied about the moment where I would have to answer to the Power-that-be for being still alive. 'What an aggravating twist of fate!' I was thinking, waiting for Round Two.

At night I could not sleep despite the medications I had been given. By that time I had realized that I was in a hospital, but the chaotic environment was oddly confusing. I could hear people screaming and arguing constantly, staff and patients shouting alike as if no one was in control. It felt strange because though my head was a bit wobbly, I could vaguely remember that hospitals usually feel like places of safety. Besides, on the following day I still had not been told what I was doing there. I could only figure out I had been brought in for stripping in broad daylight, and certainly it did not feel good.

I have been brought up with principles and most of the time I can say I have good manners. I have never wanted or tried to flash my knickers in a bar for money, let alone my naked bottom on the high street for free. I was not drunk or under the influence of any drug when the ambulance picked me up. I knew from living in South London for nearly a year that it is not exactly Eden. So what on earth was I thinking when I started walking naked down the road? I was not thinking. I felt an urge, as if I had no choice. I obeyed the numbers on the front door which instructed me to do it. As I was walking I heard a voice, possibly my mother's, saying: 'Trust. Don't worry.'

On the second evening in hospital a compassionate nurse finally told me what I so eagerly needed to know. She was a mature African Caribbean lady whose name was ironically Mercy. 'There is no need to be afraid,' Mercy said as she sat down on my bed where I was sobbing loudly. 'You're in a psychiatric hospital and for the time being we are going to look after you.' Her soft voice made me feel better and words slowly started to make their way towards my mouth again. She kindly explained that I had been brought to an acute psychiatric ward; a safe place where people came to when they were unwell and at risk of hurting themselves. All this would have made perfect sense without the heartbreaking screams of a patient being forcefully restrained next door.

'A psychiatric hospital?' I replied, slowly recovering my speech. 'I don't want to stay here. I want to leave. Right now!'

'I'm afraid you cannot leave at the moment,' she said with a supportive smile.
'Why?'
'Because you have been sectioned. You are under Section 2.'
'What does "sectioned" mean?'

'It means you cannot leave this place unless the doctor says so. But don't worry: you'll be just fine here. We are going to take care of you.'[1]

Dear Mercy, she had good intent. I was grateful to her for reassuring me; for telling me I would be OK, for explaining it was only a temporary situation. That was all I needed at that stage but no one else had bothered giving me an introduction to the ward.

I cannot precisely remember when I was duly assessed for the first time. I can only remember that during a preliminary assessment that probably took place during the first 24 hours, I chose not to disclose my real identity. I borrowed a friend's name, address and past. I was scared someone would come and get me in hospital to punish me for eluding my premature death. Also, I must admit, it felt great pretending to be someone else at the time.

They were not giving me any medication during the day but would insist that I took a few tablets in the evening. When I asked nurses what these were actually for it was very hard, not to say impossible, to get an accurate or satisfying answer. 'Just take them!' I was being told evasively, with smiles dangerously filled with teeth. I had been told they were 'antipsychotic' medications. I had no idea what it meant but I can assure anyone whose mind is broader than the paradigms of medical science that I did not need them because my mind felt clearer then than it had ever felt before, or since. Crystal clear.

I was not talking much and maybe, as the remaining senses of blind people intensely develop in order to compensate for their absent sight, I suddenly found myself endowed with some sort of a psychic ability. I felt I could read people's minds and communicate with them telepathically; especially with the dead and other spirits. Of course, the medical model dismisses this kind of testimony and rather turns it into a delusional symptom usually associated with schizophrenia. But it cannot explain everything.

A few months before I was in hospital I had developed a fascination for numerology. In a nutshell, numerology sets principles according to which quantities – hence, numbers – shape the universe and everything in it including us. The ripples of cosmic dynamics can be felt positively or negatively depending on our willingness to acknowledge their impact and, if necessary, to modify our behaviour consequently. From a sceptic's point of view (for whom no evidence will ever suffice) it may be seen as one more informal science often vaguely associated with esoteric beliefs. However, to people with no lid on their mind who are aware that there is more out there than what we can see, numerology has the potential to provide valuable – and they soon realize, accurate – answers.

I have learned to keep under firm control my fascination for this attractive way to investigate past, present and future but at that time, it had become an obsession. I could not see several digit numbers without compulsively making endless calculations maybe leading to extreme actions (e.g. door numbers persuaded me to take my clothes off) or astoundingly revealing but frankly scary interpretations.

On my first assessment, instead of answering doctors' questions about my mental state, I told them the world was in grave danger and they had no idea about the changes that were about to take place. As they were prompting me, I told them about a new world order – thousands of people – men, women and children of a same nation were about to die as a result. I talked about storms and floods: the sea coming out of its bed to swallow mobs on the shore, cities floating on grubby waters; wrecked. I told them these planes recently hitting the Twin Towers were only for starters but I decided to stop there because I could see they clearly were not ready for the main course. They were fidgeting on their seats, nervously. Looking back at world events that have since occurred, maybe they could have paid more attention to or shown a bit more empathy for my 'psychotic' discourse. They did not take me seriously. They smiled at me with wry sympathy and increased the length of my compulsory treatment. No doubt I would be on the ward for a while: as far as they were concerned, I was completely bonkers.

In 48 hours I had displayed a variety of symptoms which from the medical model's perspective could have been associated with schizophrenia, bipolar or personality disorder – or a combination. It may be that none of the doctors involved in trying to establish my diagnosis wanted to take responsibility for admitting that such labels are in most cases utterly irrelevant. Whatever the reason, they first settled on 'clinical depression'. This seemed to me to be startlingly inconsistent with the textbooks on symptoms. Is a woman who wanders naked in the streets, is convinced she experiences thought interference, hears voices, is obsessed with punishment and claims she is someone else, just *depressed*?

To be fair to them, as my 'treatment' progressed the doctors did not completely dismiss the diversity of my symptoms though they obstinately associated them with some sort of pathology. Especially when I said I could drink a man under the table and was daily self-medicating with cannabis because so far I had not found any other strategy to survive my futile and horrible life. I was secretly hoping they would help me tackle my long-term addictions but they did not. Instead they triumphantly concluded on a second diagnosis: 'drug-induced psychosis'. This is what they wrote into my medical records for I have fortunately seen them since. Go and try to get a decent job after that.

Meanwhile, most patients were nice to me. I was listening to them, they were listening to me. We had no one else to talk to, really. Nurses were always too busy; some of them used to carefully avoid me, maybe because I gave them 'the look' when they talked to us in a defensive or patronizing way. They were scolding us as children. Luckily most of the time we would see nurses only for lunch and medication time because, apart from Mercy, they would cluster continuously in their poky office.

As for agency staff, the supposed 'care' assistants, it seemed the majority of them could not care less about people's distress. It seemed as though they would intervene only if they could foresee an opportunity to exercise their limited institutional power. Most of the time they were completely idle; they just watched TV or read the newspapers. It was virtually impossible to tell who was staff and who was a patient if they were sitting next to each other.

If people were threatening to slice each others' throats they would stand up unwillingly with a big sigh, raise an angry finger and lecture the renegades about hospital policies. Not that qualified staff seem to remember their peaceful conflict resolution or de-escalation training either. Eventually they would come out of the office, only to bark at patients and threaten them with forced injections: usually no attempts were made to resolve quarrels to ensure they would not resume later. So, naturally, they would.

I believe 90 per cent of these conflicts could have been avoided if staff had talked more, and more calmly to patients in the first place, but they were always too busy with paper work. I think some of them would have liked to spend more time with us if they could have done so. They were just doing as they were told but sadly, judging by their behaviour, they were also told that being kind is a sign of weakness.

During the second assessment, I gave doctors my real name and talked about my past. I was beginning to make sense of some conscious and subconscious patterns I knew were involved with the punishment I had imposed on myself when I stripped naked. I talked to them about my mother's suicide when I was a child, and about the guilt I felt most of my life for thinking I had failed to be a good enough carer. I explained to them how a few weeks before I was admitted to hospital, a close friend of mine died of cancer. She had let me stay at hers when I moved to London, had been like a mother to me. Her death had profoundly affected me and somehow revived the shock and memory of my mother's death.

I told them in confidence that the voices I could hear were the voices of the dead because the people I loved kept dying around me all the time since I was a child. The doctors were scribbling frantically as I was talking but did not look convinced. They did not ask how I felt about my missing father, my violent uncle, the absence of support from my family, or why I had been mainly raised by my godmother. Oddly, it did not seem to occur to them that my childhood traumas had had any impact on my recent behaviour whatsoever. At the time it made me feel angry and upset but I have since then observed that this is the way the medical model tends to work.

REFLECTIONS ON THE MEDICAL MODEL AND THE USER PERSPECTIVE

About three years ago a friend of mine tried to maim his private parts after experiencing a series of unusual and unexplainable circumstances which led him no choice but to act the way he did. He was arrested in the backyard of a priest who was trying to dissuade him from slicing off his own penis. The priest called the police, who brought my friend into hospital. Soon afterwards, his sister and I went to visit him where he was detained and asked to see his doctor. The doctor thought my friend had schizophrenia and should remain on medication for the rest of his life. We explained to him that in the past my friend had been repeatedly sexually and physically abused; first at school and later by members of his local church. The severity of his self-harm obviously had a lot to do with not having had the opportunity to talk about the guilt and shame which both the child and the adult had repressed. His sister, who had some experience of distress herself, insisted that he be referred for talking therapy.

His doctor scornfully laughed at us and said psychiatry was not concerned with this kind of lyrical nonsense. We thought our attempts had been in vain, but a few days later my friend found the courage to tell his doctor things he had never told anyone before. He knew his distress and the past were inextricably linked. Still, the doctor did not take any of it seriously but simply increased his medication. Such is life. If those doctors who systematically dismiss patients' opinions were to admit that some of them – though they are medicated and detained – have strong and valuable insight, they would have little or no grounds to section them.

I have been told by some mental health practitioners outraged by my experience of acute services that these places are far better nowadays than they were back then. Yet, I was commissioned by a Mental Health Trust to undertake an audit on acute wards in 2008 and, from what patients told me, they are not much better off than I was seven years previously. Service users contributing to Chapter 7 make similar points. There have been some improvements, yes, especially with the physical environment. However, in a health care culture where targets and 'payment by results' seem to have become the main tools for assessing and dealing with people's feelings and emotions (considering the little time mental health and social care professionals are allowed to spend having 'one-to-one' with their clients) enabling individuals' Recovery is likely to remain an intricate challenge. In addition, 'sometimes so much fear and frustration have been aroused in the ill person that fixing the breakdown does not quiet them. At those times, the experience of illness goes beyond the limits of medicine' (Frank 1991, p.8).

Many theorists have tried to grasp what lies behind the medical model's reluctance to value service users' opinions about their own illness and furthermore, about the concept of illness altogether:

> There is a struggle point going on in the mental health field to fix the meaning of 'consumer participation' as 'representation', something which would incorporate it into the dominant liberal political discourse... It is those practices which 'unsettle' the comfort of mental health professionals in their relationships with psychiatric consumers/survivors. (Bannerji *et al.* 1991, quoted in Church 1995, p.73)

Acknowledging patients' perspectives has at least two implications. The first one is the necessity for professionals not only to look at their practice but also to look at their own fears, feelings and contradictions, and above all, assumptions. The two following quotes demonstrate that some professionals are aware that it can be an issue for many of their colleagues, with very understandable reasons.

> In my experience the primary defence used to prevent power sharing and authentic communication stems from professionally constructed judgments about the validity and meaning of the users' experience of mental distress and their perceived competence. Many professionals really believe they know what is best for their patients. I have observed consistently the professionals' defensive need to separate and maintain a secure base of identity, status and power. This defence appears to activate because of anxiety and fear when facing emotional distress or pain. Many staff seem unprepared

> emotionally to engage on a deep level that resonates with the users' experi-
> ence of being in the world and are conditioned to split off and rely on pro-
> fessional constructions of what is happening. (Bertram 2002)

The benefits of taking into account patients' perspectives in their own
care and treatment have been increasingly acknowledged since the early
1990s. The User Movement had paved the way for this in the 1980s but
I don't think people saw any significant change in practice before the
1990s. Many practitioners recognize that we are 'experts by experience'
therefore entitled to participation and recognition, but this can be highly
challenging for some professionals. It may remind them of the necessity
to address their own mental health issues and the distress we all come to
experience, at some point, as human beings.

> Consumer participation has the potential to call mental health professionals
> to account not just for how we do our work but for who we are. We should
> expect this process to be painful and conflictual... We need to get inside the
> dynamics of our conflicts in order to learn more about what is going on.
> (Church 1995, p.74)

Thus, the more professionals will be tuned into their own feelings the
more equipped they will be to respond to patients' distress, and to care
for them: 'Empathy builds on self-awareness; the more open we are to our
own emotions, the more skilled we will be in reading feelings' (Goleman
1995, p.96).

Another implication of acknowledging clients' perspective is that it
enables people who have been stigmatized and often disempowered to
hold services and professionals accountable for their decisions. By doing
so we regain some independence, indirectly reclaim a social status and
critically shift the balance of power. This is a major issue because historically psychiatry has been and potentially remains a powerful tool of control. The collusion between psychiatry and Nazi Eugenics and its use to
silence dissidents in Communist Russia in the early twentieth century are
well known and painfully documented. In the wrong hands, psychiatry
can be and has been used to shape society according to the requirements
of the dominant social class.

Corrigan (1987) pointed out that we all hold ideas and experience a
variety of social relations which are not always in accord, and may even
clash, with society's dominant ideologies. Such autonomous experiences
and beliefs, when held by people who are mentally distressed, often form
a distinct repertoire of knowledge, leading holders to be described as
'noncompliant' because their views frequently conflict with what are considered 'socially acceptable' models.

In a thousand quiet, implicit, prismatic forms (this different repertoire of knowledge) does become communicated through *particular* social relations... Given a different eliciting context it can be vocalized, concretized and, above all, acted upon. (Corrigan 1987, p.23; emphasis added)

Hence, society in general is not ready for 'mad' people's opinion to be credited or valued: many people would have no choice but to face and question their own distress, which is always painful. As for the medical model, psychiatry is not ready for patients to help shape the understanding of the world because, in fact, there would be very little need for its coercive power in such a world (only 3% of mentally ill people are known to be violent). No need to silence, medicate or restrain those who 'disrupt the rational' where rationality is no longer imposed as the norm.

WHY USER INVOLVEMENT?

Involvement means patients (i.e. clients, service users, consumers, survivors) becoming involved in their own and others' care, at individual or service level.

It is clear that I would never have felt such a blazing need to become involved if the care and treatment I had received in hospital had been appropriate or suitable. Nor would I have so actively sought and found ways to manage my mental health if I had not experienced what it feels like to be detained, deprived of most of my civil rights and yet, not supported. Having considered the mental health system as a whole, I would not have tried to contribute to change if change had not been so manifestly needed. Deep down, I could feel that going through this ordeal was not a complete waste of time. I could occasionally hear my mother's voice saying softly: 'Trust. Don't worry.'

My involvement started in hospital because reduced to the loneliness and at times the despair of seclusion, one is ineluctably drawn to the essential, that is, to survival. Only years later did I become strongly aware of involvement's political dimension and its potential to oppose oppression of the weak and the deprived.

Five days after my admission my mental state seemed to have greatly improved. I had given up on the Gandhi role; my boyfriend had brought me some clothes. (Without my permission, staff had contacted him when I revealed my address and identity.) Constantly hungry, I was swallowing hospital processed food in industrial quantities. I enjoyed the meals. They were the only moments where people interacted, so I made them last. There were no occupational or therapeutic activities on the ward:

I was dead bored. There was nothing to do apart from watching TV; reading was not an option because medication's side-effects were making it impossible to concentrate. Dwelling in this nihilism was threatening to put my sanity at risk so I started to write about what I was witnessing; the showers full of vomit or diarrhoea we could commonly enjoy in the morning, the 'care' assistants, the way patients were treated by staff and, often, neglected. I was fascinated for instance by the process of putting highly distressed patients on what was called 'close observation'. It was definitely *observation* only; no communication was involved. I believe therapeutic *engagement* was not yet valued at the time. It was maybe seen as the fantasy of scholars whose opinion was little valued by some ward managers, many of whom were qualified and competent administrators who could balance spreadsheets and budgets but did not seem to have much understanding of interpersonal skills. Since then I have observed when sitting on recruitment panels as an independent consultant that the people who hire them do not always consider this to be an issue. So understandably, from those managers' perspective, plain observation rather than genuine engagement was usually seen as the best answer to people's distress.

For example, one woman who was an expert in foul language was being regularly watched like a monkey in a cage. It would infuriate her. Staff used to twiddle their fingers or read the newspapers in front of her bedroom door while she spun round in it endlessly. None of them would talk to her, so she would retaliate with loud and abusive monologues everyone else had to endure. It was hard to get some rest then because she knew an awful lot of ways to use the f... word. Expecting to get better in such an environment was indeed a mere delusion. Other patients like my roommate were restlessly shuffling up and down the corridors all night, desperately trying to get hold of a rarely granted cup of tea. 'If we do it for one, we will have to do it for everyone', a curt nurse told me once. However, staff policy consistently highlights the importance to treat everyone as an individual. This idea held by unhelpful staff that individual care is a luxury is an example of the ludicrous gap which sometimes splits policies from practice.

> Most people who deal with ill persons do not want to recognize differences and particularities because sorting them out requires time. Even to learn what the differences are, you have to become involved. Generalities save time. Placing people in categories, the fewer the better, is efficient; each category indicates a common treatment: one size fits all. (Frank 1991, p.45)

So my first experience of involvement was to start writing about many missed opportunities to treat people with dignity. About bad and sometimes good practice, though good practice was occasional rather than something you could rely on. Not much was done to contribute to patients' well-being apart from nurses accidentally crossing the 'us and them' boundaries because they were themselves depressed, or angry at the management. And I also noted the helpfulness of nursing students saturated with ideas about 'patient-centred care' in a system that would not allow it.

Deep down I was boiling with rage and praying one day someone would give me the opportunity to let the whole world know what this 'soothing place of safety' really was. At the time I was at war with the universe, true, but I was even more furious and appalled with these institutions and individuals who were supposed to protect vulnerable people but would contribute to their distress instead, and were being paid for it.

In order to write my little reports I had no choice but to ask nurses for paper and 50 A4 sheets later the rumour was spreading that I could be a spy. The doctors must have been told I was up to no good because two days later I was summoned unexpectedly and told I was going to be discharged... on the same day.

The doctors asked me how I was doing, with crocodile smiles. I carefully replied that I was feeling OK as far as my own self was concerned but was aware some people had a raw deal. They were genuinely intrigued. I told them people should be treated better, like human beings, not animals in cages. I suggested a few things I thought would help people to recover since these things were usually making *me* feel better. On this occasion I do not know if they listened but I was discharged two hours later.

WITHOUT A DISCHARGE PLAN

The doctors and other people involved in my care wrongly assumed I did not need any benefits (i.e. the welfare allocation for incapacitated people) or follow-up care because at the time I was living with my boyfriend: another assumption with yet more sore consequences. In fact I decided not to stay at his any longer because voices were telling me to sort myself out without his help. I also became increasingly worried he would stab me in my sleep. He was not that bad but I had reasons to be paranoid. Strange things were happening. The TV was switching itself on without me using the remote control. Occasionally the little icons of my mobile phone's wallpaper were spinning erratically.

At the same time highly positive but just as inexplicable phenomena were daily unfolding. My actions and thoughts were guided by benevolent spirits who would show me right from wrong and intervene when I was in trouble, or at risk of being hurt. I could see 'signs' everywhere which I was able to read like an open book.

It is not my concern if medical science and many people dismiss the existence of other realms or realities. I do not believe, I *know*, the dead – family and friends – protected me during the only period of my life where I found myself homeless.

I had no money and nowhere to go because I did not want my friends to see me distressed. I tried to go to shelters but they would all tell me that I needed a referral, and I did not have one. I slept here and there: on benches, in buildings' entrances. It was cold. I can never look at a homeless person the same way since. There is nothing to develop compassion like the memory of aching. One night I tried to sleep in Brixton police station but they did not let me. So what if another exotic cuckoo was camping on the pavement? It was none of their business. Brixton cops are hard to impress... Not surprisingly, ten days later I was back in hospital.

This time round the police brought me in. They restrained me as I was screaming and struggling to run away from my boyfriend's clutch right outside his home: he would not let me go. No one was bothered about what could have been domestic violence. Yet worried that blood could be shed on their front door, the neighbours called the police when I fell on my back, surrendering to a convulsive fit during which I saw a white angel smiling at me with his arms open.

The police treated me like a criminal and laughed at me because I was hysterical and dishevelled. So did hospital staff when I begged them to take me in because 'signs' and numbers had become strikingly overwhelming. Back on the ward I was convinced staff also wanted to stab me so that patients could have me for dinner. No more belly-burst feasts: I would hide under my bed during mealtimes. I was experiencing what I imagine animals feel when they are led to the abattoir, a horrible sensation that made me consider becoming a vegetarian from then on. At the peak of these delusions, I was so scared I tried to grab a nurse's hand for comfort and begged her in tears not to leave me alone. She took her hand back and angrily commanded me to go to my room until I could remember my manners.

I spent Christmas there. The nurses gave me a Teddy bear. I loved it. They also gave me a forced injection to prevent me from breaking my skull once I was banging my head against the wall: I guess it was easier than holding my hand. Just when hope was starting to give place to an actual form of psychosis, another patient came to my rescue. X was kind and compassionate to me: he turned the tragedy into a joke by making fun of rude nurses and deriding the desolation in which we were left. Peer support is often undervalued by mainstream services, as Humphrey Greaves points out in Chapter 4, but without X there is no doubt I would have been driven completely insane.

To the doctors I told nothing but lies this time: I knew the only way to get out was to play the 'reality' game and to say I was fine. Consequently I was rapidly discharged and came out of an acute ward for the second time in January 2002 with only one but firm intention: never to get back in again.

CONCLUSION AND GOOD PRACTICE GUIDANCE FOR IMPROVING INPATIENT CARE

- Inpatients need to be more involved in their own care, more informed of treatments and have more options, e.g. type of (or option to refuse) medication, access to talking therapies. Information relating to individual and diverse needs, including spiritual needs, should be formally acknowledged within one week of arrival on the ward.

- Increased communication between staff and inpatients has to become a priority, and not only through schemes such as 'Protected Time'. It must be actively promoted by team leaders and managers on an ongoing basis.

- Service users must be involved in delivering training on this and other issues impacting on their Recovery. Comprehensive training for nurses on communication and interpersonal skills must become compulsory and core to the programme.

- Inappropriate staff behaviour and attitudes need to be tackled through effective supervision (including agency staff). Formal appraisal should include performance indicators duly addressing this current shortfall.

- Ward based community meetings ought to be more effective and where possible user led. They should aim to improve relationships between staff and patients as well as practical matters, such as quality of the environment.

- Service users who have had appropriate training should be involved in setting standards for and undertaking regular external reviews in order to help address gaps in service delivery and standards of practice.

- Therapeutic activities (whether occupational, educational, vocational and/or artistic) need to be actively facilitated or increased on the ward for these are indispensable to the therapeutic environment as they are to Recovery.

- Inpatients should be better informed of their legal rights when detained and be able to access effective and independent advocacy services. Notices displayed on the wall cannot be seen as 'providing' information.

NOTE

1. In the UK people deemed to be at risk of hurting themselves or others and who are suffering from mental distress can be compulsorily detained in psychiatric hospital under the Mental Health Act 1983. Section 2 is an assessment order lasting up to 28 days.

REFERENCES

Bannerji, H., Carty, L., Dehli, K., Heald, S. and McKenna, K. (1991) *Unsettling Relations: The University as a Site of Feminist Struggles.* Toronto: Women's Press.

Bertram, M. (2002) 'User involvement and mental health: Critical reflections on critical issues.' *Psychminded*, 15 December. Available at www.psychminded.co.uk/news/news2002/1202/User%20Involvement%20and%20mental%20health%20reflections%20on%20critical%20issues.htm, accessed on 12 May 2009.

Church, K. (1995) *Forbidden Narratives: Critical Autobiography as Social Science.* Amsterdam: Overseas Publishers Association.

Corrigan, P. (1987) 'In/forming schooling.' In D. Livingstone (ed.) *Critical Pedagogy and Cultural Power.* South Hadley, MA: Bergin and Garvey.

Frank, A. (1991) *At the Will of the Body: Reflections on Illness.* Boston, MA: Houghton Mifflin.

Goleman, D. (1995) *Emotional Intelligence: Why It Can Matter More Than IQ.* London: Bloomsbury.

Sen, D. (2006) *The World is Full of Laughter.* Brentwood: Chipmunka.

CHAPTER 6

The Road to Recovery

Aloyse Raptopoulos

An exile am I in this world.
An exile am I, for I have traversed the earth both East and West,
Yet I found not my birthplace, nor one who knew me or had heard my name
(…)
And no man understands the language of my soul.

('The Poet VIII', Kahlil Gibran)

INTRODUCTION

Following on from my breakdown and hospitalization described in Chapter 5, I will now describe the process of taking my Recovery into my own hands and how becoming actively involved helped me to find a sense of purpose and fulfilment in my life.

Out of hospital I had no choice: I had to find a cure for my life – easier said than done. In the words of Brown (2008):

> We do have a choice about what happens to us... More choice is important in making sure that you can get the help that you really need, but it does put more responsibility for our well-being into our own hands. (Brown 2008, p.4)

I found this to be brutally true when I decided to stay clear of the mental health system. In fact, I was nowhere near out of it. After my second hospital admission I was referred to a Community Mental Health Team (CMHT), this time in accordance with my discharge plan, and was prescribed medication by a psychiatrist whom I had to meet every two weeks.

Until then I was convinced psychiatrists were just careless control freaks because I had never had a chance to meet a considerate one, but at the CMHT two of them genuinely tried to help. They wrote letters to my tutors (at the university in Canada, who gave me extensions to finish my masters dissertation). It is regrettable that both these doctors had to leave after six months because of the rotation system they were on as junior doctors. This meant that as soon as a therapeutic relationship was starting to develop between us, they were gone. I saw three or four different doctors and each time I had to tell my story over and over again. It was draining and humiliating because there are things one can hardly say once without feeling ashamed, even if there is no reason to be. Still, I can say that when coercive treatment is not their priority, there are some well-intentioned practitioners in this profession like in any other: they are just hard to find, and even harder to keep.

INVOLVEMENT BRINGS THE SUSTAINABLE RECOVERY THAT MEDICATION CANNOT PROVIDE

Medication, nonetheless, is a topic we never managed to agree on. Medication is widely – though arbitrarily – seen as the cheapest and most efficient treatment by general practitioners (GPs) and psychiatrists alike. However, I can say from personal experience and from what peers and other service users (see Chapter 7) have told me that medication is not most people's preferred and *informed* choice. Regrettably, it is often the only treatment offered.

While in hospital I observed what I consider to be truly unethical practice with regard to medication. I felt for a 14-year-old girl detained on my adult ward who was given nearly 40 tablets a day – a handful at each meal. Any form of Recovery for her must have been or will be a highly demanding challenge.

At first, I was prescribed anti-psychotic medications combined with antidepressants. When I started to take them I was cautious because I had struggled with damaging habits in my twenties but, hoping to get better, I thought: 'It's legal, it won't kill me!' However, after three weeks I began to notice subtle, and less subtle, changes in my behaviour. My cognitive functions slowed down to the point that spelling a simple word became significantly hard work. I could no longer make decisions. I became idle and revelled in lethargy all day long. Nowadays I do not have much time to watch TV but back then I would remain 'glued to the box' for hours without having any idea of what I was watching. When you are on medication, it is not easy to have the kind of belief in your and other people's dignity that is needed in order to get back in control of your life. Standing up for yourself or for others is a struggle because your motivation is numb. Standing full stop may actually be an issue.

As a matter of fact, the physical side-effects were no less demeaning. Antidepressants gave me palpitations similar to panic attacks and increased my anxiety. Anti-psychotic drugs stunned me as if I had been severely hit on the back of the head. I could not read or write, which was certainly an issue since I still had a 40,000 word dissertation to write in order to complete my masters degree.

More ominously, I had no feelings whatsoever. I felt like a vegetable rotting in a glass jar through which no emotions would come in, or out. Anyone could have settled comfortably in my head and made himself at home; I surely would not have noticed. There are many descriptions by service users about the damage unsuitable medications can do to one's life – for example:

> It is important to give the person suffering the distress the choice about medication. I remember being given Stelazine and as a result of its sedative qualities, I could barely keep my eyes open. My psychiatrist pointed out my psychotic symptoms diminished under Stelazine, but did he really expect me to live the rest of my life like as a zombie? The medication got rid of my psychotic symptoms – and my life too. We are more than just psychiatric symptoms and labels. Anti-psychotic drugs don't give you a meaning to life. They just calm you down enough to make it slightly easier to find one. (Sen 2006, p.96)

I asked my consultant to change my medication. I wanted my brain back, and so he agreed to prescribe me new ones. A few weeks later I was sitting on the toilet when I suddenly felt paralysed from head to foot and thickly fell on my bathroom floor with my trousers down my ankles. Feeling my right cheek on the cold tiles I was at once perfectly aware that this was not an ideal location and position to recline, but I could no longer move a finger: my brain's coordination seemed to be entirely gone. I could not say how long I lingered there without any control over my body but when I finally managed to get up and stumble out of my bathroom I was shaking with fear.

I planned to stop taking medications if it meant ending up in a wheelchair at an age where others are trekking the world and dancing their legs off. Who knew what could have happened in the future? Doctors said medication had different effects on people. One thing I knew for sure is that I did not like the effect it had on me.

I find it deplorable that psychiatrists and many other mental health practitioners appear to believe that drugs, sometimes in very high doses, will bring about actual and sustainable Recovery when in my experience, and that of many people with mental distress, they do not. In many cases, it can at best suppress symptoms. At worst, people are so sedated they forget who they are and what has kept them alive so far. Common practice can even be harmful:

> This practice of immediately going for a drug to relieve a symptom reflects a widespread attitude that symptoms are inconvenient useless threats to our ability to live life the way we want to live it and that they should be suppressed or eliminated wherever possible. The problem with this attitude is that what we call symptoms are often the body's way of telling us that something is out of balance... If we ignore these messages, or worse, suppress them, it may only lead to more severe symptoms or more serious problems later on. (Kabat-Zinn 1990, p.277)

I know some people could not sleep, handle daily activities and manage their symptoms on the whole without medication. At times I wonder if it would not make my own life slightly easier to get back on them. Yet, I have lived enough to say that without an occupation, a hobby or a passion bringing meaning to one's life, tablets alone bring only temporary – and possibly deceptive – relief. Freud himself is said to have stated about medications: 'Their job was to transform neurotic or psychotic misery into ordinary human unhappiness' (as quoted by Sen 2006, p.106).

Medication's inadequacy to improve my mental health and the possible damage it could do to in the long term meant I had to try to develop my own coping mechanisms but side-effects were preventing me from relating to what some people dare calling the 'real' world. So I stopped taking my medication despite my consultant's vehement objection, promising me I would go back to hospital if I did. His attitude was unfortunate as his support would have made it safer. I had been warned by peers that stopping all at once would expose me to severe withdrawal symptoms (often mistaken for 'relapse'). As I progressively reduced my medication's dosage my mood, will-power and energy notably shifted. I was beginning to understand that more often than not, people know far better than anyone else what is good for them.

RECOVERY NEEDS THE SKILLS AND KNOWLEDGE GAINS THAT INVOLVEMENT PROVIDES

I also know from personal and now professional experience that people often rely on medication because they have not been encouraged to consider whether engaging in an occupation like volunteering might

effectively stimulate and help to sustain their Recovery. Reinforcing occupational therapists' familiar perspective, the evaluation report of *Capital
Volunteering* produced in 2008 by London's Institute of Psychiatry brings
additional evidence that volunteering is a highly efficient Recovery tool:

> Participants identified the following key areas in which they had experi-
> enced direct gains from taking part: improved well-being, personal and
> social development, practical skills and knowledge, employment skills and
> experience, volunteering achievements, supportive environment and a sense
> of achievement in helping others. (Bellringer, Easter and Murray 2008,
> p.8)

I was certainly eager to engage in any social or educational activity but felt
like my prospects for development were rather thin, both personally and
professionally. I spent 2002 struggling to complete my dissertation for my
masters in sociology of arts. I was still highly distressed but it provided me
with some of the skills I needed to make sense of myself, society and the
world we live in. However, in terms of employment, visual arts fit in a very
specific domain where the people you know are often far more important
than what you know yourself. I had no contacts in the art world and felt
like a lost soul 'drifting and drifting, like a ship out on the sea'.

I was struggling to find my own identity. Not knowing my father,
having lost my mum at an early age and feeling rejected by members of
my family had a lot to do with the murky state of mind I maintained for
many years. My godmother had done her best to provide me with love
and education but when I went to live at my uncle's house I felt like I had
no one I could rely on. At times, I felt disincarnated, disembodied.

After my hospital admissions, my psychiatrist and other professionals
then involved in my care had firmly stated that I was not well enough to
go back to employment. At first, I was temporarily housed in a hostel and
– on my vigorous request – put on to a waiting list for talking therapy.
Later on, my social worker found me a flat which gave me the core stability I needed to think about what I could do with my life: volunteering
seemed to be the best option. The desire to contribute to my peers' well-
being (and need I say to my own) led me to register on a course for aspir-
ing volunteers facilitated by my local Mental Health Trust in June 2003.

I did not know then what impact this initiative would have on my
life. It was only two years later, when I was invited to join the Capital
Volunteering Project Board, that I realized how my decision to go and
volunteer my time and services had been at the time the best I could
have made. Set up in 2005, Capital Volunteering was a three-year pan-
London project aiming to reduce social exclusion by creating volunteering

opportunities for people experiencing mental distress. Its evaluation report (Bellringer *et al.* 2008) has brought additional evidence that volunteering, and any form of involvement in occupational, artistic, educational or vocational activity, helps people to rebuild their lives, and significantly helps to acquire or extend the personal social network some of us desperately need to feel socially included:

> participants had made friends through Capital Volunteering [CV]. For some this was their first opportunity to make new friendship groups and for others this was a novel experience. CV had provided the opportunity to revive old or unused skills. For some the project had also allowed them to pursue past interest and occupations... the opportunity to apply creative ideas and skills. The emergence of new skills and knowledge were identified in a variety of areas ranging from music to computers to mental health... CV had provided valuable work experience and an opportunity to prepare for employment for [X number of] participants. They viewed their volunteering experience as a stepping stone back into work and as a 'halfway house' in the process of obtaining future employment. (Bellringer *et al.* 2008, pp.9–11)

Through voluntary involvement, I was going to gain and achieve all of the above: as part of my volunteering course in 2003 I had to undertake a mental awareness training, which I thoroughly enjoyed. Noticing my enthusiasm the trainers suggested that I might join them at the Lambeth Mental Health Promotion Unit (LMHPU) based at South London and Maudsley Mental Health Trust (SLAM). They said I could help with writing their quarterly newsletter and become involved in delivering training.

INVOLVEMENT PROVIDES THE SUPPORTIVE ENVIRONMENT RECOVERY NEEDS TO FLOURISH

Today still, LMHPU's aim is to inform local and highly diverse communities about mental health issues and services. Back then, they used to invite people experiencing distress to participate in staff training and to help spread awareness in schools, an activity discussed by the Jewish Care service users in Chapter 8. This was an effective way to tackle stigma and for teenagers to see that 'mad' people were not really mad. I was grateful to the trainers to have been given a chance to do something I considered useful instead of being depressed at home.

Towards the end of 2004 I started to provide a 'service user perspective' in staff training for SLAM with the SUITE (Service User Involvement in Training and Education) unit. The two people managing the unit were service users themselves and could relate to my concerns. Both of them were very skilled trainers from whom I learnt a great deal. Encouraged by their support I kept co-delivering staff training for statutory agencies including local rehabilitation and social services on an ongoing basis. At the same time I was carrying out all sorts of other involvement tasks: providing a client perspective on Trust committees aiming to improve care and treatments, delivering talks in conferences and awareness events, sitting on staff recruitment panels, etc. Participating in staff recruitment was refreshing because I was still recovering from using acute services and knew what staff skills and attributes were needed in order to deliver decent care.

Through involvement I was also invited to become a judge on Clinical Governance and Excellence awards panels; the former highlighted best practice and the latter recognized doctors' achievements. As an independent consultant I still do this work today and must admit I find profound satisfaction in marking and ranking application forms from consultant psychiatrists. Ethically, I rely on the forms' content and use my judgement to do so, not my memory. However, where I see inauthentic statements, or no evidence of patient-centred practice, I keep in mind the people whose lives rest in doctors' hands for I used to be one of them.

In 2005 I started a nine-month 'Training the Trainers' course and went on other courses in order to add theory and qualifications to practice. I was convinced that using services had provided me with valuable expertise but I was not sure yet of how to put my own message across. The opportunity to become a professional trainer presented itself in 2006 when Mental Health Media invited me to deliver their anti-discrimination training course for service users. In order to be shortlisted, one essential criterion was to have personal experience of distress and discrimination. It increased my confidence to be appointed *because*, and not *in spite*, of who I was.

Training peers rather than staff was a turning point: I thoroughly enjoyed it because I felt I could contribute to their own empowerment by teaching them how to tackle the stigma we commonly experience. It was also refreshing not to have to justify myself for being a patient as, when I was teaching staff, my capacity was occasionally challenged. In October 2006 I was told that a senior lecturer at London South Bank University (LSBU) was looking for people who wished to use their experience of using services to teach mental health and social care students, another opportunity I did not miss.

Helping to teach at university was an exciting prospect but additionally there were growing pressures for me to go back to full-time employment. I had moved from benefits onto a 'permitted work' scheme, allowing me to receive some financial support and to work at the same time, the little money I earned being deducted from the benefits received. However, this transition period had reached its limit. I would soon find myself with no resources because from the benefits' perspective, the fact that I was so actively involved meant that I was perfectly fit for full-time work. No one specialized in mental health at my job centre so they could not figure out that involvement was my main therapy: that it was a means to heal, rather than an end (to earn money). So even though I knew the university would not give me a full-time job I was hoping I could start accumulating enough paid work to become self-sufficient.

At LSBU I became involved in student learning and recruitment. The lecturer I was practising with immediately made me feel at ease: she talked to me as if we were equal and kept referring to me as her 'colleague', which was decidedly encouraging. I learnt I had something to say, something students could make use of. By working with and observing her and other senior lecturers, I found out how I wanted to say it. The support, trust and respect they placed in me gave me the confidence I needed in order to believe in myself again, and to ascertain the teacher I always wanted to be. I soon realized that teaching students was different from training staff or other adults. It required some skills I did not have so I enrolled on a Post-Graduate Certificate in Higher Education (PGCHE) the following year. My personal tutor and course director have had a lot to do with the pleasure and interest I regularly took in class.

INVOLVEMENT IN TALKING THERAPY: AN ESSENTIAL COMPONENT OF RECOVERY'S HOLISTIC APPROACH

Regular involvement did not mean I stopped experiencing distress but my anxiety significantly reduced. As for my severe and enduring depression, I had the chance to address it in psychotherapy, which has done wonders for me. What a shame that I had to wait one and a half years to be assessed.

Together with practising involvement at a service level, involvement in my own care, powerfully encouraged by my psychotherapist, had a significant impact on my life. He would not say much but when he talked, words of wisdom poured out of his mouth. A very kind man, my psychotherapist – a very clever man too, for it is wise to be kind, not weak.

Always a little smile on his face but not a threatening smile, like doctors and nurses on the ward: a smile full of empathy and understanding.

He gave me the courage to confront my uncle for the brutality and the anguish he had put me through as a teenager (when he was my guardian). He helped me to single out the rejection of some members of my family towards me, partly because I was an 'illegitimate' mixed-race child born in Africa but raised in France in my mum's white family. It is not pleasant to experience jealousy and discrimination from people you love: my psychiatrist taught me to stop looking for love where love cannot be found.

I became actively involved in my treatment and Recovery through our weekly partnership work. I can say 'work' because therapy is no rest and does feel at times like a full-time job, but it was worth it. I would not be able to manage my mood swings and anxiety today if it had not been for making some sense of the guilt, frustration and anger triggered by the upheavals of my earlier life. Nonetheless, talking therapy is not always a success.

When my psychotherapy came to an end after 18 months I felt saddened and unsettled by the split with my therapist, who had become such an important part of my life. Besides, I knew I still had the need for addressing personal issues and for the professional support that can be found when people are lucky enough to access *effective* specialist services. I requested to be put onto another waiting list.

Many months later I was admitted to a different service and started seeing a new therapist, who did not make it clear at first what *psychodynamics* was about, and what the process would be. I know I should have done some research myself and I make no excuses for my naivety. I had read that psychodynamics was a form of talking therapy closer to psychoanalysis than to psychotherapy, and I foolishly thought I had an idea of what it was about. It turned out that I did not; however, the therapist was definitely more of an issue than the therapy in itself.

In a few words, psychodynamics is a model essentially based on the relationship between the therapist and the client. 'What if they do not get on?' you may think, as I certainly did. Well, this would be due to 'the *client's* struggle with relationships and possibly to his incapacity to form any'. I do not know if this is what psychoanalysis promotes but that is what my therapist spat at me when we had our first argument.

In contrast with my previous psychotherapist, who facilitated my wholehearted involvement, she seemed to try to do everything in her power to sabotage it. She used to indulge in the kind of damper that practitioners lean on when they are incompetent by claiming that I would not 'engage'. Now, it is obvious that *engagement* must necessarily be a two-way process: services and professionals have the responsibility to engage with their patients as much as patients are expected to engage with them. Alas, the timing of my weekly appointment did not suit my agenda, which was pretty full by then. I had just become self-employed and could not afford to turn down job offers. I explained that another time or day would have been more convenient but it was not negotiable. I was made to feel deeply uncomfortable when I had to tell her that I would miss a session because of work: it became a permanent worry on my mind. Services were not flexible enough to facilitate my engagement but she would make me bear the burden. Mediocre practice, poor judgement...

She used to do another thing common to professionals whose training gets in the way of spontaneous and open understanding: she would attribute my display of natural or basic emotions to pathologies. For instance, if during a session I became upset, irritated or visibly angry because she would persist to put in my mouth words I had not said or meant, I was immediately said to be 'aggressive, inconsiderate and ungrateful'. How was this supposed to make me feel better? She had no interest in my job's progress, or in the gratification and stability that I would reap from it. She would pay attention to my emotions only when I was in tears and tatters, only *then* would I engage! Yes, a bad therapist can do a lot of damage. People turn to them when they feel vulnerable and as the saying goes, *with great power come great responsibilities*: she simply did not keep up with hers.

INVOLVEMENT REDEEMS SELF-ESTEEM AND ENABLES POSITIVE LIFESTYLE CHANGES

Being involved in my and others' care prevented me from feeling useless. It bestowed on me a sense of purpose; it taught me what it means to have and take responsibility. It also provided me with a grounding routine and a balanced lifestyle which I never really had before. Fleeing my uncle's violence when I was 16 meant that in order to sustain my exile from France, I had been waitressing in catering and bars most of my life: night life does not usually provide a balanced lifestyle. I became increasingly convinced that I could contribute to make my immediate environment a better place. People I worked with anyway seemed to think or say so and this belief stimulated my potential for learning and growth. Through sustained involvement I increased personal awareness, developed capacity and acquired a valued role and status (to my view anyway) boosting my confidence and self-esteem.

As part of my coping strategies I realized how much I could influence the way I felt by maintaining personal discipline, and by *exercising* regularly. Everyone has different needs and resilience but as far as I am concerned, I know I must get up early, do breathing exercises and meditation, talk to spirits, avoid drinking during the week and drink in moderation when I do, eat well (what has not been killed) and get enough sleep, otherwise my mind will be weakened and unbalanced. In 2004 I started doing yoga to stabilize my mind, and kick-boxing to release my anger, both helping to address the stress we are all likely to accumulate. I now often work 15 hours a day but I make time for classes in the evening at least several times a week. I also take a little run from time to time, if only to remind me that I must stop smoking cigarettes.

I mentioned in Chapter 5 that, having no awareness of medication before I went into hospital, I had self-medicated with cannabis for years. Involvement even helped me to get rid of that habit because I needed my brain for the tasks I was carrying. A statutory meeting when on cannabis is a lost battle and, as a service user representative, I wanted to be trusted and reliable. Teaching or training does not allow mind digression, especially not the kind of detour that a chronic habit demands of one's cognitive and nervous system.

After years of constant smoking, it took time before I could sleep and eat properly without it. Luckily, even in the evening I had to do a lot of writing for work so there was no time for it and, gradually, I weaned myself off the desperate need to avoid contact with my own feelings. Usually people know they are busy when they need a diary to manage all their appointments. I already had a diary but realized I was working 80 hours a week (fuelled by mania, cyclic depression and anxiety) only when I became too busy to smoke my brain off. Some of these symptoms still remain but I have learnt to control the distress they used to cause me and have found meaningful ways to put them at use, so turning a problem into an advantage.

CONCLUSION

Involvement is one of the most efficient therapies someone with mental distress can undertake for and by him- or herself: it is way more effective than medication, and it is a lot safer. It is about professionals and service users working together to improve the quality of care people receive, and to widen choice. Choice enables people to lead a healthier and happier life *according to their individual circumstances*, the core principle of Recovery.

In my view, involvement is also a social and political activity that must take great care not to become complacent and sanitized. In order to help in bringing about change, we service users or former service users have to be assertive enough not to let go of our opinion in favour of the loudest speaker: the voice of the institutions.

We may face the criticism of those who dismiss involvement because they are reluctant to share some of the power that has been taken away from us, and to admit that mistakes are only human. Thankfully many professionals and academics – like those who supported me with my Recovery – are aware that, by partnership alone, services (and to my view, society as a whole) can be improved. Despite the system's inconsistency they are doing their best to enable this collaboration, and lead by example.

Through experience I have come to know that Recovery has little to do with the end of medical symptoms and the clinical interventions thought to make them disappear. Recovery means being able to survive the consequences of past ordeals and to overcome the negative feelings these have imposed on us, so that we can make the best of what we have now. We cannot change the past but we can take some responsibility for the way we feel and act towards it now. Ultimately, this is the only thing over which we really have any control.

Recovery is achievable even for those who suffer severe and enduring distress as long as professionals, students and members of the public help people to identify their goals and support them in finding their own ways to achieve their potential.

As for me, I am still on the road.

GOOD PRACTICE GUIDANCE FOR EFFECTIVE USER INVOLVEMENT

- Involvement at individual level is barely an option: no one should hand over their life to professionals on a plate. It should not be assumed that people do not have capacity because they are not compliant (HM Government 2007a).

- Service user involvement in service planning and delivery is definitely not an option: it is a statutory expectation for all UK health and care agencies and professionals (see, for example, Department of Health 2006; HM Government 2007b).

- Accordingly, more training (to enable the service user's contribution), time (to enable professionals and academics to provide sustained liaison and support) and resources should be allocated to facilitate the involvement process.

- Involvement at service level is effective only if both parties – clients and professionals – value each others' opinions and share the decision-making power. If not, it is likely to remain tokenistic and undermined by protocols.

- Involvement in higher education is not only beneficial but also necessary. Service users can and must perform a variety of tasks, e.g. providing input in courses and curriculum reviews, sitting on advisory groups and committees.

- Peer support is underestimated: those said to be vulnerable can gather significant strength through unity with peers. Often, peer support can help us to make sense of our distress way better than any diagnosis would do.

- People should be proud of using or having used mental health services, not ashamed. The world is full of individuals who are not officially ill but struggle with their lives. Attempting to address personal issues that some misleading media call 'madness' is in fact the first step towards sustainable autonomy.

REFERENCES

Bellringer, S., Easter, A. and Murray, J. (2008) *A Pathway to Recovery. A Qualitative Study of the Impact of Capital Volunteering in Participants' Lives*. London: Health Services and Population Research Department, Institute of Psychiatry, King's College London.

Brown, M. (2008) 'Change and choice' (Editorial). *One in Four*, Autumn.

Department of Health (2006) *Our Health, Our Care, Our Say: A New Direction for Community Services*, Cm 6737. London: The Stationery Office.

HM Government (2007a) *Mental Capacity Act*. London: The Stationery Office.

HM Government (2007b) *Local Government and Public Involvement in Health Act*. London: The Stationery Office.

Kabat-Zinn, J. (1990) *Full Catastrophe Living: Using the Wisdom of your Body and Mind to Face Stress, Pain and Illness*. New York, NY: Delta.

Sen, D. (2006) *The World is Full of Laughter*. Brentwood: Chipmunka.

CHAPTER 7

User Involvement in their Own Treatment and Care

Jenny Weinstein with service user colleagues

INTRODUCTION

User involvement in their own treatment and care is perhaps the most vital element of the Recovery approaches discussed in this book. Enabling individuals to have some choice about the treatments and therapies they receive and offering holistic, reliable, but flexible support systems are crucial to promoting Recovery (Brown and Kandirikira 2006). The role of the professional is no longer simply to 'treat' the person and 'make them better' but to provide the person with information options and choices to enable them to take control of their own condition and to deal with issues such as employment, relationships, leisure and living conditions (Barnes *et al.* 1999; Shepherd, Boardman and Slade 2008).

The term 'user involvement in treatment' can mean different things to different stakeholders (Fischer *et al.* 2007). For service users, the most important aspect is often about feeling that they are listened to and understood by mental health professionals; medical professionals are more likely to see user involvement simply in terms of informed consent to drug treatment, while other professionals such as community or residential staff focus on the active participation of service users in the particular treatment programme(s) offered by their services

For the authors of this chapter, user involvement begins with genuine choice and empowerment. Drawing from the literature and from the experiences of 16 service users,[1] some named and some who chose to be anonymous, this chapter will explore the concepts of choice and empowerment and consider whether and how these concepts are put into practice in acute settings, medication management and community care. It will end by discussing the government's strategy to enhance choice and empowerment through its personalization agenda.

CHOICE

The NHS modernization agenda (Department of Health 2000) was all about patient choice but many mental health service users remain sceptical about what they perceive as the rhetoric of choice. This may be explained by the possibility of compulsory treatment remaining as a shadow hanging over them (Perkins and Repper 1998) or by the history of poor mental health practice, stigma and not being taken seriously that has undermined their trust in the system (Prior 2003).

Although the number of people compulsorily detained under the Mental Health Act 1983 is small in relation to the total number of mental health service users, the stigma of being in hospital 'under section' has a disproportionate impact on how patients perceive mental health services, how professionals perceive patients, and how the public perceives mental illness (Rankin 2005). There is an analogy to be made with the small number of children who are taken into care against the will of parents and the powerful impact that this group has on how children's social services are perceived by service users and the public. The fact that professionals have recourse to legal powers to intervene can undermine users' belief that they hold any genuine rights to make their own choices. For this reason the extension of compulsory powers through Community Treatment Orders that were introduced in the Mental Health Act 2007 were bitterly resisted by service user groups (Batty and agencies 2007).

The importance of choice has been recognized in many countries such as Australia, New Zealand, UK, USA and Canada, where national strategies are beginning to employ the language of patient empowerment, involvement, participation and choice (Sainsbury Centre for Mental Health 2006). According to the UK government, 'Better health care outcomes are achieved when…both patient and health professional share in making decisions about treatment and care' (Department of Health 2004).

Our Choices in Mental Health (Care Services Improvement Partnership (CSIP) 2006, p.5) sets out the government's vision in more detail and identifies four key areas where service users want more choice:

1. Choice about how they live their life

2. Choice about how to contact mental health services

3. Choice about when and where a mental health assessment is undertaken

4. Choice of treatment and care options.

A study undertaken by the Sainsbury Centre for Mental Health (2006) found some examples of government guidance being put into practice but also many settings where traditional approaches were barely disguised and service users did not feel they had any real choice. Many service users, especially those from Black and Ethnic Minority backgrounds, appear to be confused about what choice could actually mean for them on a day-to-day basis (Sainsbury Centre for Mental Health 2006). In some cases it has been difficult to change the culture and attitudes of entrenched and powerful mental health professionals but, in the main, the problems seem to revolve around resources. Without a range of affordable, culturally sensitive and appropriate services from which to chose, the principle of 'choice' remains somewhat academic.

There are some who would argue that choice and Recovery models may be like 'The Emperor's new clothes' – people are afraid to ask the awkward questions which may include:

- How helpful is choice when someone is really ill?

- What information and support are required to enable people to make informed choices?

- What happens when a health professional honestly believes that the patient's choice is not in their best interest?

- To what extent should the views of the main carer be taken into account if they conflict with those of the service user?

- Who is responsible or accountable if agreeing to the service user's choice leads to further difficulties?

While not denying the relevance of addressing these issues, there are a number of straightforward 'choices' that have been consistently expressed by service users (Faulkner and Williams 2005; Shaping Our Lives 2003; Wallcraft 2003) that would not pose complex ethical dilemmas although they would require a change of mind-set. For example, service users have been requesting more talking therapies (BBC News 2007), 24-hour access to sympathetic crisis support, more women-only services, more support with social problems such as parenting, benefits and housing, a

financial safety net for people wishing to return to work and more culturally competent mental health staff (Weinstein 2008).

More radical commentators regard 'choice' in mental health care as
meaningless without far-reaching changes. For example, Linnett (2003), a
service user, thought that current approaches to service user involvement
are 'simply an elaborate way of leaving things as they are'. He asserted
that tinkering with existing services on the basis of user feedback is
tokenistic when the services themselves are not fit for purpose. A service
user (SU) who contributed anonymously to this chapter expressed similar
views from her experience:

> The fundamental problem of much existing mental health care de-
> livered via the so-called 'medical model', as I see it, is that it takes as
> its point of departure existing resources and treatments. These may
> have been tried and tested but are rarely fully evaluated for how ef-
> fective they are from the perspective of the patient – a party often
> mute or rendered so sometimes because of the treatments or the
> nature of their illness. Worse still, the assumption can be, and in my
> case has been, 'she simply doesn't know what she's talking about'.
> Times, in the frighteningly recent past, when I have attempted to ex-
> press my emotional distress, it has been simply written off as 'symp-
> tomatic' of my diagnosis, thus adding to my distress. As a consequence
> some treatments have lead to deterioration rather than an ameliora-
> tion of my condition. (SU anon)

Other user co-authors had varied experiences of whether choice was offered that seemed to depend on attitudes of individual professionals:

> Not always for myself. I now thankfully have a very understanding GP.
> (SU anon)
>
> I am quite fortunate my CPN [community psychiatric nurse] is always
> ready to listen to me and cater to my needs. (SU anon)
>
> I only see my GP, not mental health people. He is only interested
> in the medication. He is not interested in other ways of treating my
> mental health problems. (Giulia)
>
> [It]…depends on who your care manager is and their perceptions/
> prejudices. (SU anon)
>
> It does depend on the kind of relationship you have with your psy-
> chiatrist. (SU anon)

Others stated that they were often not offered any choice about their medication.

> Not always, often told what we need as regards to treatment – very oppressive! (SU anon)

> If you are discussing your care with them and you disagree with their suggestions, they think you are getting ill again. (Sheila)

Users differentiated between experiences in hospital and the community, feeling that they were listened to more in the community and supported in making choices about their lives.

> At least they don't restrict how you live your life. (Sharon)

EMPOWERMENT

Empowerment may appear to be a self-explanatory term but in health and welfare discourses, its meaning is contested (Gomm 1993). Social workers and mental health nurses are taught that they should 'empower' their service users but if professionals are 'empowering' service users, this implies that the professionals are holding the power and are 'giving' (some? all?) away to the users. In this process, there is a sense in which the professionals are deciding how much power to offer rather than acknowledging full rights and equality of service users.

In the words of an anonymous SU contributor to this chapter:

> Empowerment is the key if done right! Pros cannot empower others… A big mistake in thinking. The users/survivors need to be given the support, space, understanding, trust to empower THEMSELVES! (SU anon)

Thompson (2005) suggests that in order for service users to gain full equality and exercise their rights, professionals must help to equip them 'for the challenges of tackling the social disadvantages and equalities they face. Empowerment is not only a psychological process but a social and political one' (p.125).

> Empowered to me means having a say, being given the right information to make informed choices. (SU anon)

The above definition offered by a SU contributor is supported by Rethink (2008). Its policy states that for too long, people with mental health problems have been 'subject to the views and decisions of people who think they know what's best for them...empowerment enables people to take charge of their own lives and is a key component in recovery' (Rethink 2008, p.1).

Some users had experienced this approach working well:

> I find my support worker invaluable as she encourages and empowers me to make informed choices about my life. (SU anon)

> I think that the culture of a place is what promotes empowerment. (SU anon)

Others were more cynical:

> I used to hear this word all the time in care/community but do not really see this in action. (SU anon)

> No, I don't see it. I try to empower myself. I don't rely on the so-called professionals. (SU anon)

> It's hard to feel empowered when taking psychiatric drugs. (SU anon)

ACUTE SERVICES

There is frequently a degree of resistance expressed in the classroom about the possibility of user involvement in the inpatient setting. The argument goes that people are on the ward because they are unwell and they need and want to be looked after; they are not in a state to make their own decisions. Even admissions to hospital wards where they are treated for physical health problems can make people feel powerless and rapidly institutionalized. Like the authors in Chapters 3 and 5, mental health service users often apply words like 'terrified', 'humiliated', 'bewildered', 'no one told me anything', 'no one listened to me' to describe their experiences of being in psychiatric hospitals. While there have been significant improvements in some inpatient units (Star Wards 2008), feared features of the 'old regime' still exist such as:

- a violent atmosphere where tensions rise and someone lashes out

- absence of a sense of safety

- an institutional environment with locked doors everywhere and staff jangling bunches of keys

- limited run-down communal areas

- people having to queue up for their medication

- staff avoiding contact and communication unless it is coercive or about administering treatment

- physically able bodied people being cooped up indoors with very little opportunity for fresh air and exercise

- institutional food that does not take account of religious and cultural needs

- racism and/or lack of cultural awareness

- mixed gender areas where women are physically or sexually harassed

- very limited choices of activities

- no access to talking therapies

- no interest in or support for the person's life before or after entering hospital, e.g. family relationships, housing, benefits or employment (Hardcastle *et al.* 2007; Laurence 2003).

Service users' comments on their experiences in hospital included the following:

> The environment is noisy with people kicking off. It makes you feel worse not better. (Sheila)

> You can get up whenever you want but if you get up late you miss breakfast, which is only out till 8. (Sharon)

> There are activities. You put your name down on a list. I remember there was toy making. (Sheila)

> You could go out but only if there was a member of staff to go with you and they don't often have time. (Sharon)

> I have bipolar and I was getting high. They put me on an older people's ward because I am over 65. Everyone else had dementia. There were no activities at all – just the TV. (Geoff)

A service user writing about inpatient care (Janner 2008, p.3) says that 'personal autonomy' is critical for patients on mental health wards. She finds that exercising choice helps people to regain self-esteem which, in turn, aids Recovery and that:

there is little that is less conducive to feeling in control of our situation than fear of actual violence... Personally, I am much more scared at the prospect of coercive treatment (being forcibly injected, wrestled to the floor, stuck in a 'seclusion room') than being biffed by another patient. (Janner 2008, p.3)

An anonymous co-author agreed:

> It is the worst possible scenario and usually the worst possible environment...you just want to get out as quickly as you can. I find wards intimidating – not restful. (SU anon)

Certainly, for service users in hospital, what makes the most positive difference to their sense of well-being is the sense that they are being listened to, that relevant information is communicated clearly to them and that there is the potential to make trusting relationships with staff and other patients (Gilbert, Rose and Slade 2005).

In response to service users' demands, an initiative called Star Wards has been established to encourage the staff on inpatient units to improve communication and environment. Service user involvement is central to the changes so that ex-patients participate in the recruitment and selection of staff, patients are involved in the day-to-day running of the ward, patients chose the activities they would like to do, patients are involved in the development of their care plan and hold their own copy. The importance of talking therapies is accepted so all patients can expect some one-to-one time each day with their key worker. All religious festivals and fete days of service users are celebrated and care is taken with customizing meals to individual diets and cultural preferences. Support is offered with phone calls, benefits and housing problems; flexible visiting hours enable family to visit; staff are accessible to family members and training on leadership is made available to service users, carers and volunteer advocates (Star Wards 2008).

These changes have led to the following reported improvements:

- Patients are more involved with their treatment and recovery, enjoy better relationships with staff and each other, and discover new skills and interests.

- Carers are appreciative of their relatives' mental health treatment and daily activities.

- 50 per cent of pilot sites had a reduction in violence.

(Star Wards 2008)

Improvements suggested by service user co-authors include the following:

- More information, more choice. (SU anon)

- Yes, it can be improved drastically by knocking it down and demolishing the system. (SU anon)

- Better access for smoking and other freedoms. (SU anon)

- Yes, a listening ear would be useful. (SU anon)

- More better trained staff. (Geoff)

- Staff who mingle with the patients. If someone goes on the rampage the staff hide in the office. (Sheila)

- A crash pad for evenings and weekends. If I am unwell there are places I can go in the day but I need somewhere safe for evenings and weekends. (Sharon)

- Home Treatment is a good alternative to hospital but you can't always get it even if you ask. (SU anon)

MEDICATION

User perspectives below set the scene for discussion in this section:

I was on melaryl and it suited me. The psychiatrist decided that there may be a risk of physical disease – I think it was something to do with heart – and he put me on olanzapine. It was awful. I put on three stone in six months and I was so demoralized. The psychiatrist did not only refuse to listen to me but he refused to listen to the dietician who was working with me. (Sharon)

They [my CPN] was trying to tell me what medication I should be taking and what dosage. But I told her that the particular medication they wanted me to take did not agree with me. So they changed it to one that was more suitable for me. (SU anon)

Unfortunately the psychiatrists and CPNs are too worried about risk to allow patients to have a say. (Geoff)

I think there should be more emphasis on helping people cope with less medication as the side-effects are more heinous than symptoms they are supposed to control. (SU anon)

> We're not allowed a say – prefer alternative remedies i.e. herbals and homeopathy, exercises and complementary health treatments. (SU anon)

Medication is clearly a key issue for both service users and mental health professionals and it is often the focus of conflict between them. Although there have been significant improvements in the efficacy of drugs to alleviate mental distress, there are still a number of unresolved problems that cause reluctance in many service users to take their medication or in the language of the professionals to make them 'non-compliant'. According to the *Oxford English Dictionary*, 'compliant' means 'tending to be excessively obedient or acquiescent' or 'complying with rules or standards'. The continuing use of this terminology by mental health professionals is unlikely to persuade service users of professionals' genuine commitment to concepts of choice or empowerment.

The side-effects of many drugs reduce the quality of life of service users, for example making them feel restless and unable to concentrate, drowsy and apathetic, giving them the shakes, causing them to slur their speech, leading to weight gain and/or lack of sex drive. It is therefore not surprising that when service users begin to recover from their mental distress, they are keen to reduce or stop the drugs that are having these effects. Inevitably, for some service users, stopping their medication leads to a recurrence in their illness thus undermining progress towards Recovery.

It is therefore absolutely essential that service users and practitioners discuss the treatment options, including the side-effects, dosage, possible alternatives and longer term implications of any treatment plan. Service users who make informed decisions about their treatment are more likely to make a good Recovery because they feel in control of their own care plan. On this basis, the National Institute for Health and Clinical Excellence (NICE 2002) guidance recommends that any decision regarding treatment should be arrived at jointly with the professional.

This should be straightforward but mental health professionals who were surveyed in this regard expressed their commitment to user involvement in principle but found that limited resources, dearth of service options, strict agency criteria, lengthy administrative procedures, and statutory requirements can be barriers to making this a reality in practice (Fischer *et al.* 2007). A risk averse culture is also a barrier to genuine user involvement (Davidson *et al.* 2006), especially in acute or residential care. Mental health services in the community seem to offer more scope for responding to service users' requests for modifications in their treatment or support with practical aspects of their lives. Nevertheless, according to Pemmaraju and Patel (2007) the user involvement movement had made a difference between 1992 and 2005 with service users now feeling more involved and informed, although more time still needs to be offered by doctors and nurses to explain and discuss the potential side-effects and treatment plans with all their patients.

COMMUNITY CARE AND THE PERSONALIZATION AGENDA

Background

The Prime Minister's Strategy Unit (2007, p.33) report describes personalization as 'the process by which services are tailored to the needs and preferences of citizens'. The personalization agenda originated in user-led campaigns of the 1970s such as the independent living movement and the social model of disability and has been influenced by the practical work of a consultancy called In Control, which pioneered the use of self-directed support and personal budgets as a way to reform the current social care system (Carr with Dittrich 2008).

Care Programme Approach (CPA)

The notion of person-centred care began to take shape in services for people with learning disabilities (Department of Health 2001) and became the benchmark standard expected for all care groups and consequently was required to underpin the Care Programme Approach (CPA) for people with mental health problems (Department of Health 1990; NHS Executive and Social Services Inspectorate 1999). In a number of surveys investigating service user involvment in CPA, users reported varied experiences (Carpenter et al. 2004; Hounsell and Owens 2005; Warner 2005); those who felt that they had been fully involved enjoyed a higher level of satisfaction and better outcomes but a significant minority either did not know about their plan, had not signed or received a copy and did not know their care coordinator. Care plans are genuinely person-centred only when they holistically address service users' social issues such as employment, benefits, housing, leisure and relationships and not just the dosage and timing of their medication (Weinstein 2008; see also Tew 2005). A service user contributing to this chapter pointed out that even when they were involved in the care planning process, the agreed plan was not always implemented in practice.

Direct payments

Direct payments are cash payments made to individuals who have been assessed as needing services, in lieu of social service provisions. Taking control of their own funding enables service users to employ their own personal assistants so that they are not dependent on agency workers who arrive at inconvenient times or are inflexible about the tasks they are prepared to undertake. Instead of having to attend established day centres, service users may use the 'day care' element of their social services funding to undertake an activity of their own choice such as a computer class, visit to the leisure centre or theatre outing.

Direct payments are now available to all adult service user groups although take-up by people with mental health problems has been very low (Davey 2007). There may be a number of reasons for this. First, direct payments relate only to the social services care element of a needs assessment while, as emphasized by one of the anonymous service user commentators, mental health care should be holistic with health and social care needs integrated:

> My question is why, at a time of my life when I am feeling more vulnerable than ever before, am I subjected to endless referral and assessments? I would like to have been treated holistically and as a person going through a period of huge emotional distress. (SU anon)

Second, insufficient information was made available about the scheme, therefore many mental health service users and even mental health professionals were unaware of this option. Just over half of the service users involved with this chapter had heard of direct payments and/or personalization and their responses were mixed:

> The reason I know about it is that I was assessed for a direct payment by my social worker a while ago. I decided to spend the money on a personal assistant to help me in the house and I set up a separate bank account to manage the money and everything. I was then told that they had decided that the assessment was wrong because it was my own social worker and it should have been someone independent. They said I was not eligible. After all that, I just did not have the energy to appeal. (Sharon)

> Yes – I think it is a good idea. (SU anon)

> Yes, but I still remain to be convinced that it is going to work. (SU anon)

> Changed the name to confuse us – is it a good idea? Not really. (SU anon)

A third problem has been the attitudes of mental health professionals who have been sceptical about the ability of people with mental health issues to manage their own payments. This is particularly problematic as support and advocacy – an essential part of making the scheme viable – tend to be very scarce.

Personalization

Building on the philosophy of person-centred care and direct payments, the government's extended 'personalization agenda' is now set to revolutionize services for adults including people with mental health problems. It aims to ensure that every person across the spectrum of need will have 'choice and control over the shape of his or her support, in the most appropriate setting' (Department of Health 2008).

The new programme was trailed in the government's Green Paper *Independence, Well Being and Choice* (Department of Health 2005) and fleshed out in the White Paper *Our Health, Our Care, Our Say* (Department of Health 2006). This White Paper was celebrated as one of the first documents to fully join up health and social care in its strategic vision. Sadly, when it came to implementation, separate guidance was published in a document focused only on adult social care (Department of Health 2007) while what was needed was a coordinated health and social care implementation strategy.

Nevertheless, the proposed outcomes coincide very closely with many of the demands of mental health service users. People will be helped to:

- live independently

- exercise maximum control over their own life

- participate as active and equal citizens, both economically and socially

- have the best possible quality of life, irrespective of illness or disability

- retain maximum dignity and respect.

(Department of Health 2007, pp.2–3)

Individual Budgets (IBs)

One of the limitations of direct payments, as indicated above, is that they replace only services funded by Social Services. Individual Budgets (IBs) were piloted and evaluated to explore the potential for pooling a number of funding streams such as Supporting People and Access to Work from which the individual could chose to take cash or services or a mixture of both. Unfortunately for all adult service user groups, NHS funding is excluded.

The explanation for the exclusion of NHS resources is the constantly recurring intractable problem that means-testing, charging and eligibility criteria would remain as part of the resource allocation system (RAS) for IBs where NHS services remain free at the point of delivery. An evaluation of the IB pilots (Glendinning *et al.* 2008) found that even the pooling of those funding streams that had been included in the resources for IBs proved quite complicated causing numerous legal, financial and account-ability barriers which frustrated practitioners.

The pilot sites developed their own RAS, often based on the In Control model (Waters 2006, p.4), which involves service users being invited to undertake their own self-assessment using a simple format to identify their own needs:

1. Looking after myself – my personal needs

2. Relationships

3. Being part of the local community

4. Work, leisure and learning

5. Making decisions

6. Staying safe from harm

7. Complex needs and risks

8. Family carer and social support.

Glendinning *et al.*'s (2008) evaluation found that budgets were most often used to purchase assistance with domestic chores, social, leisure and domestic activities. However, there were examples of more creative uses such as the purchase of a pet to assuage loneliness or the purchase of a car for someone whose fear of public transport had previously kept him at home. Nevertheless, where the service users' individual requirements led them to wish to spend the money in less conventional ways, such as to use their full year's leisure allowance on a two-week holiday, officials were unclear about boundaries and criteria. Although take-up was low among mental health service users for reasons outlined above, those who did hold their own budgets expressed strong feelings of satisfaction about the control they felt that they had regained over their lives (Glendinning *et al.* 2008). Mental health service users were the group most likely to use IBs to purchase services that were not associated with social care such as gym membership, help from a personal trainer, aromatherapy or training in a new activity such as pottery or photography (Manthorpe *et al.* 2008).

George, a service user who had been involved in one of the IB pilots, described at a seminar (Doubleday 2009) how an individual budget had improved his life. After 20 years of living with mental health problems he was offered £1000 instead of services. At the time, his psychiatrist was recommending a period of respite care. Instead of paying for this, he decided on a cheaper option and went to Tunisia for his first holiday in years. As this left him with change and he is keen on art, he bought some art materials. He explained that although he could do art at his day centre, he often wanted to do it in the middle of the night when he was having difficulty sleeping. He also paid to join a dating agency, which improved his confidence, and he bought an inexpensive car that enabled him to support an elderly neighbour with mobility problems, thus enabling him to make a contribution and feel part of the community. He said that all of this kick-started his Recovery and he is now leading a fulfilling life.

While the philosophy behind the innovations is to be welcomed, as with any social care reforms, there are always significant barriers to be overcome to bring the aspirations to reality for service users and carers. Complexity of resource allocation and management of budgets could prove major impediments and, unsurprisingly, there is a concern that the government's motivation may be to cut costs. This was a fear expressed by some of the service user contributors to this chapter, who were concerned that services such as their local Drop In Mental Health Centre would be cut in order to pay for the IBs. The centre offers a cheap nutritious lunch, a warm friendly environment, relaxed, optional activities and support from staff and fellow members. Co-authors expressed concern as to whether a group of service users, even if they pooled their IBs, would have enough money to pay for this kind of resource in the future. Service user commentators also wondered whether the replacement of traditional services with IBs might be part of the government's agenda to get more people with a disability back to work:

> I know I could never work again. The stress would be too much. I don't mind volunteering when I am feeling better but I couldn't work. (Sheila)

Strong doubts were expressed about service users wanting to manage their own budgets:

> They would be completely overwhelmed by the bureaucracy. It would be too much for them. (Geoff)

It is envisaged that there will be an option for the social care provider to manage the IB or for the IB to be held by a trusted relative or friend of the service user indicating a need for 'trained navigators' (individuals to guide service users through the maze of service and benefits options, so that clients make their own informed choices rather than being allocated by a professional) and advocates to support IB holders whose costs may eat up any savings achieved from cutting traditional services.

Worryingly, the English legislation on direct payments does not require service users to undertake the criminal record and other safety checks on people they employ, as would be required for social care staff employed by the council or private and voluntary agencies (Lombard 2008). This means that people with mental health problems could be vulnerable to financial or other types of abuse from people they are paying to support them or to manage their budgets.

CONCLUSION

Service users are now aware that they are entitled to choice and empowerment but their experiences are mixed. More services users feel that they have choices about how they live their lives within the community than believe they are enabled to have a genuine say about their inpatient treatment. Many service users would prefer acute care to be delivered within the community via crisis houses and home treatment teams.

Although mental health professionals want to implement the new philosophy, in practice they find that they are hampered by complex bureaucratic procedures, lack of resources and the continued divide between health and social care. Service users acknowledge the difficulties imposed by systems but also find that attitudes vary among mental health professionals and that those who genuinely believe in choice and empowerment can make a difference.

The personalization agenda, direct payments and Individual Budgets are still very new to both service users and mental health professionals. Limited evidence indicates that mental health service users could benefit although there are numerous practical barriers to be overcome, crucially, the ongoing structural divisions between health and social care within Mental Health Trusts.

Genuine empowerment of service users to make their own choices will require a massive change in the mind-sets of professionals and in their perceptions of their own roles and of the strengths of service users. A major cultural shift will be required to change the ways in which professionals work if they are to become 'navigators' with a role to help service users chose their own individualized care package rather than assessors of service users' eligibility for existing traditional services (Manthorpe 2008).

GOOD PRACTICE GUIDANCE FOR INVOLVING SERVICE USERS

- Service users should be listened to and encouraged to express their views no matter how ill they may appear to be, whether they are in hospital or the community.

- Service users should not be rushed when making decisions, but should be given clear explanations of treatment requirements and procedures so that they can make informed choices.

- Service users should be given accessible written information.

- Opportunities should be made available for service users to ask questions without feeling that they will be threatened or judged.

- Interprofessional role redesign and retraining with full service user involvement will be required for all mental health professionals, to put personalization into practice.

ACKNOWLEDGEMENTS

Special thanks to service user colleagues who contributed to the writing of this chapter: Ejaeta Egoh, Sharon Hamshere, Sheila Whalebone and Geoff Worley.

NOTE

1. Ten service users responded anonymously to a postal survey sent out by Ejaeta Egoh in December 2008, one service user submitted her views in writing to Jenny Weinstein in August 2008 and four service users were interviewed by Jenny Weinstein in November 2008. Users were either members or contacts of Southwark MIND, members at Lorrimore Day Centre or members of SIMBA drop-in.

REFERENCES

Barnes, M., Harrison, S., Mort, M. and Shardlow, P. (1999) *Unequal Partners: User Groups and Community Care.* Bristol: Policy Press.

Batty, D. and agencies (2007) 'Opposition calls for new changes to Mental Health Bill.' *Guardian*, 18 June. Available at www.guardian.co.uk/politics/2007/jun/18/publicservices.uk, accessed on 12 May 2009.

BBC News (2007) 'More funds for talking therapies.' *BBC* News, 10 October. Available at http://news.bbc.co.uk/1/hi/health/7037400.stm, accessed on 12 May 2009.

Brown, W. and Kandirikira, N. (2006) *Recovering Mental Health in Scotland: Report on Narrative Investigation of Mental Health Recovery.* Glasgow: Scottish Recovery Network.

Care Services Improvement Partnership (CSIP) (2006) *Our Choices in Mental Health: A Framework for Improving Choice for People Who Use Mental Health Services and their Carers.* London: CSIP. Available at www.parliament.uk/deposits/depositedpapers/2009/DEP2009-0074.pdf, accessed on 12 May 2009.

Carpenter, J., Schneider, J., McNiven, F., Brandon, T., Stevens, R. and Woolf, D. (2004) 'Integration and targeting of community care for people with severe and enduring mental health problems: Users' experience of the care programme approach and care management.' *British Journal of Social Work 11*, 3, 281–293.

Carr, S. with Dittrich, R. (2008) *Personalization: A Rough Guide.* London: Social Care Institute for Excellence.

Davey, V. (2007) *Direct Payments: A National Survey of Direct Payments Policy and Practice.* London: Personal Social Services Research Unit, London School of Economics and Political Science. Available at www.pssru.ac.uk/pdf/dprla_es.pdf, accessed on 12 May 2009.

Davidson, L., O'Connell, M., Tondora, J., Styron, T. and Kangas, K. (2006) 'The top ten concerns about recovery encountered in mental health system transformation.' *Psychiatric Services 57*, May, 640–645.

Department of Health (1990) *Caring for People: The Care Programme Approach for People with Mental Illness Referred to Specialist Mental Health Services.* Circular C. (90)23/LASSL(90)11. London: HMSO.

Department of Health (2000) *The NHS Plan.* London: Department of Health.

Department of Health (2001) *Valuing People: A New Strategy for Learning Disabilities for the 21st Century*, Cm 5086. London: Department of Health.

Department of Health (2004) *Better Information, Better Choices, Better Health: Putting Information at the Centre of Health.* London: Department of Health.

Department of Health (2005) *Independence, Well Being and Choice,* Cm 6499. London: Department of Health.

Department of Health (2006) *Our Health, Our Care, Our Say: A New Direction for Community Services,* Cm 6737. London: The Stationery Office.

Department of Health (2007) *Putting People First: A Shared Vision and Commitment to the transformation of Adult Care.* London: Department of Health.

Department of Health (2008) *Transforming Social Care.* LAC 2008(1). London: Department of Health.

Doubleday, G. (2009) presentation at seminar on Service User Involvement in Mental Health, Anglia Ruskin University. Chelmsford, February.

Faulkner, A. and Williams, K. (2005) *Future Perfect: Mental Health Service Users Set out a Vision for the 21st century.* London: Rethink: Available at www.mentalhealthshop. org/products/rethink_publications/future_perfect_men.html, accessed on 12 May 2009.

Fischer, J., Jenkins, N., Bloor, M., Neale, J. and Berney, L. (2007) *Drug User Involvement in Treatment Decisions.* York: Joseph Rowntree Foundation.

Gilbert, H., Rose, D. and Slade, M. (2005) *The Importance of Relationships in Mental Health Care: A Qualitative Study of Service Users' Experience of Psychiatric Hospital Admission in the UK.* London: Health Services Research Department, Institute of Psychiatry, King's College London.

Glendinning, C., Challis, D., Fernández, J.L., Jacobs, S. *et al.* (2008) *Evaluation of the Individual Budgets Pilot Programme: Final Report.* York: Social Policy Research Unit, University of York.

Gomm, R. (1993) 'Issues of Power in Health and Welfare.' In J. Walmsley, J. Reynolds, P. Shakespeare and R. Wolfe (eds) *Health and Welfare Practice: Reflecting on Roles and Relationships.* London: Sage.

Hardcastle, M., Kennard, D., Grandison, S. and Fagin, L. (2007) *Experiences of Mental Health In-patient Care.* Hove: Routledge.

Hounsell, J. and Owens, C. (2005) 'User research in control.' *Mental Health Today,* May, 29–33.

Janner, M. (2008) 'Sustainable Recovery.' *Mental Health Today,* March, Star Wards Supplement Issue 1, 3.

Laurance, J. (2003) *Pure Madness: How Fear Drives the Mental Health System.* London: Routledge.

Linnett, P. (2003) 'Moving beyond user involvement.' Reproduced in *Lambeth MIND News,* Winter 2007. London: Lambeth MIND.

Lombard, D. (2008) 'Direct payment users not asking for references or CRB checks.' Community Care Inform, 3 July. Available at www.communitycare.co.uk/ Articles/2008/07/03/108688/clients-fail-to-run-crb-checks-on-pas.html, accessed on 12 May 2009.

Manthorpe, J. (2008) 'Individual budgets: Fears over transition plans.' Community Care Inform, 19 November. Available at www.communitycare.co.uk/ Articles/2008/11/19/110007/individual-budgets-fears-over-transition-plans. html, accessed on 12 May 2009.

Manthorpe, J., Stevens, M., Challis, D., Netten, A. *et al.* (2008) 'Individual budget projects come under the microscope.' *Mental Health Today 8*, 10, 22–26.

National Health Service Executive (NHSE) and Social Services Inspectorate (SSI) (1999) *Effective Care Co-ordination in Mental Health Services: Modernising the Care Programme Approach.* London: NHSE and SSI.

National Institute for Health and Clinical Excellence (NICE) (2002) *Guidance on the Use of Newer Atypical Antipsychotic Drugs for the Treatment of Schizophrenia.* London: NICE.

Pemmaraju, G.O. and Patel, D. (2007) *User involvement – Myth or Reality? A Two-point Survey (1992 and 2005) of Users' Awareness of their Treatment and Ward Milieu Preferences.* London: Priory Lodge Education.

Perkins, R. and Repper, J. (1998) *Dilemmas in Community Mental Health Practice: Choice or Control.* Oxford: Radcliffe Medical Press.

Prime Minister's Strategy Unit (2007) *Building on Progress: Public Services.* London: Cabinet Office. Available at www.cabinetoffice.gov.uk/media/cabinetoffice/strategy/assets/building.pdf, accessed on 12 May 2009.

Prior, C. (2003) *Choice, Responsiveness and Equity in the NHS and Social Care.* London: Department of Health.

Rankin, J. (2005) *A Good Choice for Mental Health.* Working Paper 3. London: Institute for Public Policy Research.

Rethink (2008) *Rethink Policy Statement 50: Empowering People with a Severe Mental Illness.* London: Rethink. Available at www.rethink.org.uk, accessed on 12 May 2009.

Sainsbury Centre for Mental Health (2006) *Choice in Mental Health Care.* Briefing Paper 31. London: Sainsbury Centre for Mental Health.

Shaping Our Lives (2003) *Service Users' Own Definitions of Quality Outcomes.* York: Joseph Rowntree Foundation.

Shepherd, J., Boardman, J. and Slade, M. (2008) 'Putting recovery into mental health practice.' *Mental Health Today*, May, 28–31.

Star Wards (2008) *Star Wards at a Glance Guide in Full Colour.* Available at http://starwards.org.uk/?page_id=8, accessed on 12 May 2009.

Tew, J. (2005) *Social Perspectives in Mental Health.* London: Jessica Kingsley Publishers.

Thompson, N. (2005) *Understanding Social Work: Preparing for Practice*, 2nd edn. London: Macmillan.

Wallcraft, J. (2003) *The Mental Health Service User Movement in England.* Policy Paper 2. London: Sainsbury Centre for Mental Health.

Warner, L. (2005) 'Review of the literature on the Care Programme Approach.' In Sainsbury Centre for Mental Health (ed.) *Back on Track?* London: Sainsbury Centre for Mental Health. Available at www.scmh.org.uk/publications/back_on_track.aspx?ID=436, accessed on 12 May 2009.

Waters, J. (2006) *Creating a Resource Allocation System.* Wythall: In Control Support Centre. Available at www.in-control.org.uk/site/INCO/Templates/Library.aspx?pageid=143&cc=GB, accessed on 12 May 2009.

Weinstein, J. (2008) 'Promoting Inclusivity in Care Planning.' In A. Hall, M. Wren and S. Kirby (eds) *Care Planning in Mental Health: Promoting Recovery.* Oxford: Blackwell.

CHAPTER 8

User Involvement in Challenging Stigma and Discrimination in Mental Health

Jenny Weinstein with users from the Jewish Care Education Project

INTRODUCTION

> With mental health, the general public don't know what to say so they shun you. If it was a physical illness they would feel more comfortable. They don't understand the links there can be between mental illness and physical illness. We think about people's ignorance about mental health issues and ways to break down that ignorance. We have to show them why labels are misleading. You have to think who your audience is and how to get through to them. One thing we do is to write or speak our own testimony. This can be hard but it is very powerful in helping people understand the human being who is suffering. It's about the person – they have to understand that mental illness is not just something that happens to other people – everyone knows how it feels to be depressed. (Stan, Jewish Care service user)

Stigma was defined by Goffman (1968, p.5) as 'excluding people from social acceptance'; Goffman also pointed out how being 'labelled' could lead to stigma and discrimination. The stigmatization and poor treatment of people with mental health issues is an international phenomenon, as illustrated below by extracts from a report by Sartorius and Schulze (2005, p.7):

From India: 'My parents support me but we can't tell any of our neighbors. It would hurt my sister's chances of being married.'

From Canada: 'If I apply for the job and tell them I have schizophrenia, I won't be hired. If I don't tell them and they find out, or I suffer a relapse later, I will be fired.'

From Japan: 'Women with an illness like this will be kept at home to do domestic chores, while we men are sent out of the house.'

From the United States: 'The doctors left me waiting in the emergency room, fighting my delusions for six hours; they said other people's problems were more important.'

All over the world, we stigmatize and exclude people with mental health problems:

through blaming people for their mental health problems...shaming people for their mental health problems...not wanting to get close to them...fearing them...calling them names...talking behind their back...laughing about them...people thinking they have nothing in common with people with mental health problems...considering mental health problems embarrassing or disgraceful...thinking people with mental health problems are childlike...thinking they are unintelligent...and in other ways. (World Health Organization 2008, p.7)

The recognition of the need to challenge stigma in mental health has been a slow process, although the service user movement has been raising the issues since the 1980s (see Chapter 1). In this chapter we will briefly review some of the literature and research studies undertaken about stigma and mental health; we will consider different ways in which campaigns to tackle stigma have been organized; we will hear from Jewish Care service users about their project to address stigma and mental health awareness in their local community and we will make some recommendations about how to continue to challenge stigma in the future.

HOW SERVICE USERS EXPERIENCE STIGMA

People suffering mental distress are doubly jeopardized – first by their illness, and second by the stigma and discrimination they experience. This is well illustrated in the findings of a national survey of service users' personal experiences of stigma and discrimination undertaken by Read and Baker (1996) which achieved a response rate of just over one-third to 2500 questionnaires sent out via MIND to individuals with self-reported psychiatric diagnoses, including anxiety, depression, manic depression, schizophrenia, personality disorder, obsessive compulsive disorder, psychosis, posttraumatic stress disorder, agoraphobia, panic attacks, eating disorders, and seasonal affective disorder (SAD). The extent of the stigma they perceived is set out below:

- 34 per cent said they had been dismissed or forced to resign from jobs.

- 69 per cent had been put off applying for jobs for fear of unfair treatment.

- 47 per cent had been abused or harassed in public, and 14 per cent had been physically attacked.

- 26 per cent were forced to move home because of harassment.

- 24 per cent of parents said their children had been teased or bullied, or that they were afraid it would happen.

- 25 per cent had been turned down by insurance or finance companies.

- 50 per cent felt unfairly treated by general health care services.

- 33 per cent complained that their GP had treated them unfairly.

- 45 per cent thought that discrimination had increased in the previous five years compared with 18 per cent who thought it had decreased.

(Read and Baker 1996)

In response to a growing awareness of the impact of stigma, the government introduced the *National Service Framework for Mental Health* (Department of Health 1999) which made challenging stigma and discrimination the first duty of everyone involved in mental health services. Although this prompted discussion and action by professionals and service users, it does not appear to have had a significant impact on the day-to-day lived experience of most people with mental distress.

For example in Read and Baker's (1996) survey a respondent reported:

> Because I am labelled a schizophrenic I am treated as a second class citizen in all respects, if my label is known. My GP thinks I'm evil. (p.3)

In the mid-2000s some GPs are still not receiving adequate training in mental health, and even those who are mental health aware feel there is insufficient time to provide an adequate service to patients with mental health problems (Lucas, Scammell and Hagelskamp 2005).

In 1996 a Black patient described how:

> When I was in hospital it seemed social workers brought in new white patients, but black patients were usually brought in by the police and shoved in lock-up wards. (Read and Baker 1996, p.3)

And yet, a decade later, research shows that Black patients are still more likely to be admitted to hospital on section and more likely to be restrained (Health Care Commission, Mental Health Act Commission, and NIMHE/CSIP 2005).

Respondents to the 1996 survey reported feeling rejected by society because it was so hard to find a job; eight years later the Social Exclusion Unit (Office of the Deputy Prime Minister 2004) found unemployment rates remained at 85–90 per cent among people with mental ill health.

In 2003, respondents to research undertaken by Stanley *et al.* (2003) found that parents with mental distress continued to feel as undervalued and unsupported in their role as parents as had the 1996 respondents.

> 'I won't go back and be under any doctor or psychiatric-wise... You get branded again all over...' For this woman, contact with psychiatric services had the effect of confirming her unsuitability as a parent. (Stanley *et al.* 2003, pp.63–64)

HOW THE PUBLIC VIEW PEOPLE WITH MENTAL HEALTH PROBLEMS

Well into the twenty-first century, the general public continues to carry stereotypes about various forms of mental illness in their individual and collective subconscious. These stereotypes are regularly reinforced in the popular media. For example:

> Depression makes people useless, incapable of working and stubborn in their refusal to pull themselves together; people with manic depression are totally unpredictable and crazy; schizophrenia means split personality, hearing voices, unprovoked attacks on strangers and insanity. (See Me Anti-Stigma Campaign Scotland 2002)

In order to gain a better understanding of stigma and discrimination and to monitor progress over time, the Department of Health has conducted surveys on attitudes towards mental health since 1993. The 2007 survey (TNS Custom Market Research Company for SHIFT Media Network/ Care Services Improvement Partnership 2007) compares results with data from 1994 onwards. The sample size for the surveys has been between 1700 and 2000 adults. All of the interviews were conducted face-to-face by fully trained interviewers in the home.

Although the majority of respondents to the survey referenced above demonstrated positive attitudes, a significant minority did not and, more worryingly, some negative attitudes towards people with mental illness appear to have increased since 1994. In particular, the results indicate that younger people may be less tolerant, for example being less likely to agree that people with mental health problems should have the same right to a job as anyone else. In general, people appeared to be more likely to feel that mentally ill people could pose a threat to safety than they did in 1994, with 13 per cent more people than in 1994 thinking that people with mental health problems were 'prone to violence'.

Interestingly, over half the respondents knew someone close to them with a mental illness and one in ten acknowledged having contacted a medical professional themselves about an emotional or mental health problem. Nevertheless, ignorance about mental illness is still widespread, with respondents' most common sources of information about mental illness gleaned from TV, newspapers, films and leaflets.

This is significant because evidence has been collected (Callard 2006) to show that media portrayal of mental illness tends to reinforce prejudicial attitudes rather than to challenge them. Survey data indicated that negative stories were the most common, with murders and other violent acts perpetrated by people with mental health problems the most common news items.

Nevertheless, there have been some attempts to provide more in-depth explorations of severe mental illness using soaps or documentaries. A reality TV show (Wollaston 2008, p.27) threw together five people with mental health issues and five people without in a large castle for a few days. The idea was to identify 'who is mad and who is not'. It is pleasing to find that even the panel of 'mental health experts' were unable to accurately identify all the individuals with mental health problems.

At the time of writing, a new anti-stigma campaign called Moving People/Time to Change is being launched by a group of mental health charities led by Rethink with funding from the National Lottery. To inform the campaign, yet another survey of service users' and carers' experience was undertaken and the results presented in a publication called *Stigma Shout* (Time to Change 2008).

The *Stigma Shout* survey confirmed that stigma and discrimination is all pervasive, with close to nine out of ten service users (87 per cent) reporting its negative impact on their lives. Two-thirds have stopped doing things because of stigma and/or because of the *fear* of stigma and discrimination. These proportions are significantly higher for women, people living with severe mental illness, people who are gay, lesbian or bisexual, those with additional disabilities and the middle-aged service user population. Multiple layers of discrimination are clearly a problem, although differences based on ethnicity were not identified in this survey. Responses of users and carers indicated the following 'league table' of individuals or groups experienced as likely to discriminate against them.

DISCRIMINATORS' LEAGUE TABLE

1. Immediate family = 36 per cent

2. Employers = 35 per cent

3. Neighbours or local community = 31 per cent

4. Friends = 25 per cent

5. Work colleagues = 23 per cent

6. GPs = 23 per cent

7. Wider family = 22 per cent

8. Young people (teenagers) = 21 per cent

9. Psychiatrists = 19 per cent

10. Benefit agency staff = 18 per cent

11. Accident and Emergency staff = 17 per cent

12. Police = 17 per cent.

(Rethink 2008)

CHALLENGING STIGMA

Challenging discrimination, stigma and social exclusion has the potential to significantly improve the quality of life of those with mental health problems (World Health Organization 2008). The World Psychiatric Association's *Open the Doors* programme that operates in 20 countries, national initiatives such as *Like Minds, Like Mine* in New Zealand, *See Me* in Scotland and a host of community initiatives have been created to tackle stigma and discrimination in mental health (Time to Change 2008).

A number of models have been suggested (Sayce 2000) for helping to reduce stigma by enabling a better understanding of mental illness or by actively campaigning against discrimination. One perspective is to help people to see that mental illness is caused by biological or chemical problems in the brain – i.e. that mental illness is like any other illness so should receive the same sympathy and understanding as physical health problems. The weakness of this approach is that it does not take account of the multiple contributory causes of mental illness or the interrelatedness of social, psychological and physical difficulties. While being helpful to some extent, it is too simplistic to achieve the required change in attitudes.

Another approach regards mental health and mental illness as a continuum. This model is useful in that almost everyone is able to see themselves on this continuum and people will recognize that their own mental health will fluctuate between feelings of depression, anxiety, anger, etc. and feelings of joy and well-being. Recognizing the continuum blurs the distinction between people with mental distress and everyone else and normalizes mental illness through an understanding that it can affect anyone at some stage in their life.

Two other approaches (Sayce 2000) are related to campaigning for the rights of people with mental health problems. The more mainstream 'Disability Inclusion' model derives from the social model of disability (Oliver 1990) that requires society to change its structures and systems in order to include rather than exclude people with mental or physical disabilities. The more radical model opposes any state intervention in the lives of people with mental health problems and demands that they should be fully empowered to control their own lives and treatment.

Aspects of all these ideas have been incorporated into many of the campaigns against stigma described here. A number of organizations have struggled to find the best way to tackle the problem. In the rest of this chapter we will present and evaluate a range of anti-stigma campaigns and strategies developed in the UK.

EFFECTIVENESS OF ANTI-STIGMA CAMPAIGNS

In 2004, the National Institute of Mental Health in England (2004) produced a review of activities in relation to campaigning against stigma and discrimination with a view to determining what does and does not work. The review identified key principles that underpin best practice in mental health anti-discrimination programmes. The first encapsulates the philosophy of this book, which is that users and carers must be involved throughout the design, delivery, monitoring and evaluation of anti-discrimination programmes. There are numerous examples of user-led campaigns that are successful because the target audience learns from those who are experts by experience. For example Pinfold *et al.* (2005), investigating the successful ingredients of anti-stigma campaigns, found that

> The statements of service users (consumers) about their experience of mental health problems and of their contact with a range of services had the greatest and most lasting impact on the target audiences in terms of reducing mental health stigma. (p.123)

Some of the other findings (National Institute of Mental Health in England 2004) were that:

- *National* programmes that support *local* activity demonstrate the most potent combination for efficacy.

- Programmes should address behaviour change with a range of approaches.

- Raising awareness and changing attitudes does not necessarily lead to a reduction in stigma or discrimination.

- Programmes that aim to reduce stigma and discrimination must address discriminatory actions by individuals, groups and organizations.

- Effective approaches include social inclusion and empowerment, providing support and skills to help individuals to adapt, developing an environment of intolerance to prejudice and ensuring change is sustainable and supported by policy and legislation.

- Long-term planning and funding are fundamental to programme sustainability.

Some anti-stigma campaigns appear to have been more successful than others. In 2002 the Changing Minds campaign was established by the Royal College of Psychiatrists to end stereotypical and stigmatizing representations of mentally ill people in the media and elsewhere. The campaign's website proclaimed:

> For centuries people with mental illness were kept away from the rest of society, sometimes locked up, often in poor conditions, with little or no say in running their lives. Today, negative attitudes lock them out of society more subtly but just as effectively. (Royal College of Psychiatrists 2002)

The Changing Minds campaign funded advertisements and produced teaching and publicity materials for different audiences in different formats. However, some mental health users' groups were unsupportive of the campaign, saying that psychiatrists label mentally ill individuals for life, instead of treating them as people (BBC News 1999). It may be that service users and carers did not feel that they were equal partners in this campaign but that it was being waged 'on their behalf' rather than in partnership with them. Just as mental health service users can be stereotyped, so too can psychiatrists and there is clearly an urgent need to rebuild trust between some users and some psychiatrists (Pilgrim and Rogers 1993; Thornicroft 2006).

Service users have sometimes expressed cynicism about stigma campaigns on the basis that they are tokenistic and do not address the underlying causes of stigma. For example, a mental health activist was reported as responding to the announcement of the proposed new 'Moving People' anti-stigma campaign as follows:

> I lay a lot of the blame at the door of the government and the media.
>   It is the Department of Health and Home Office which has promoted a culture of fear and risk with emphasis on 'public protection' particularly since the Michael Stone case. (Pembroke 2007)

Nevertheless, there is some evidence that campaigns led by service users and directly using their voices can have a significant impact. One example is Scotland's See Me campaign launched in 2002, which strongly features personal stories from people who have experienced mental distress as well as support from well-known media figures and football teams. From the outset it was agreed that the campaign should:

- have a strong first-person voice

- support people with experience of stigma to be the public face of the campaign

- be direct without being shocking

- not accuse campaign audiences of being 'perpetrators' of stigma

- alert the public to the problem and win support from across a broad spectrum of society.

The See Me campaign suggests that in many respects mental ill health can usefully be compared to cancer, but, unfortunately, although the government has asserted its commitment to mental health, it has not committed the level of resources that has turned around the cancer statistics and image. When there is still so much secrecy and shame surrounding mental ill health, it takes courage and commitment for service users to speak openly about their experiences, either to targeted audiences as in the Jewish Care project described below or in the media as in Scotland's See Me Campaign.

The review undertaken by the Highland Users' Group (HUG) *et al.* (2006) four years after the See Me campaign was launched, indicates that there have been discernible improvements in the general public's awareness of and attitudes towards mental health issues with fear of mentally ill people decreasing. Fewer Scots now feel that it would be hard to talk to someone with mental health issues and are willing to acknowledge that words such as 'nutter', 'psycho' and 'schizo' are derogatory and should not be used.

IMPACT ON SERVICE USERS OF BEING INVOLVED

In previous campaigns against discrimination, it was recognized that stigmatized individuals such as Black people (Taylor and Spencer 2004, p.100) or older people (Levy 2003) often internalized the stigma associated with their condition thus undermining their own self-esteem and confidence in themselves This phenomenon has similarly been recognized among people with mental health problems:

> People with mental illness may have to recover from the stigma they have incorporated into their very being; from the iatrogenic effects of treatment; from lack of recent opportunities for self determination; from the negative side effects of unemployment; and from crushed dreams. (Anthony 1993, quoted in Wallcraft 2005, p.106)

> Eddie rejects his diagnosis of schizophrenia primarily because of the stigmatizing views held by society. He described a sense of loss and bereavement when he became unwell which he feels has prevented him from achieving his personal aspirations. (Smith *et al.* 2008, p.104)

As illustrated by Greaves and Raptopoulos in Chapters 4 and 6, a positive cycle emerges from the involvement of service users. As they become involved, their confidence and sense of well-being improve and they become more effective as campaigners. Branfield and Beresford (2006, p.11) also spoke to service users about networking and being involved:

> being involved...has given me a lot you see like I can now help people in a similar position.

Beales *et al.* (2006, pp.13–14) offer some quotations from service users about what it means to be involved:

> Has helped an awful lot, gained confidence.
>
> A chance to make a change...to the way mental health services are organized.
>
> It's helped me grow and it's great to meet people in the same situation.

In the next section users of Jewish Care's mental health services share their experiences of being involved in anti-stigma activities and discuss how this impacted on their own mental health.

JEWISH CARE EDUCATION PROJECT

Jewish Care is the largest provider of health and social care services (including mental health services) in the UK's Jewish community. The authors of this section are a team of service users, staff and volunteers keen to share their experience and reflections on the work they have undertaken together to challenge the stigma and misconceptions about mental illness within the local community and within the charity.

Jewish Care's Mental Health Education and Development Department evolved out of a dynamic interaction between service users and staff. In this team, 'user involvement' means that service users are full partners in all stages of an initiative – from the planning stage through to implementation and evaluation.

The Education Department began in an informal way. A common theme in service user feedback within Jewish Care had been the sense of rejection and prejudice from the local community in relation to mental illness. The idea of going out into the community to educate people about mental health was thought to be one way of trying to combat some of those stereotypes. Following important networking by Susan (a staff member), Susan and Stan (a service user) visited local community organizations to speak about mental health issues. The audience at one of the talks were so impressed that they asked Stan to write his testimony for the synagogue magazine. Stan recalls how it all started:

> About five years ago I was sitting in the day centre feeling sorry for myself... I spoke to Susan, one of the project workers, about how I could see nothing positive in my life and that I felt it had no purpose. Susan said she was going into the Jewish community to talk about mental illness and asked if I would go with her. I agreed and I have not looked back since.

The department now consists of three part-time staff members, one of whom is a user-employee, some volunteers and a core of about 15 users who are involved on a project-by-project basis. Some users came to the education project via other Jewish Care mental health projects. John (not his real name), who is now a key player in the Education Department, recalls:

> I had been a service user for many years but things started to change when I joined the work skills group 4 years ago. I attended every session and got interested in the employment project and the IT works. I never believed that they would be able to help me to find a job but I was roped in as a volunteer administrator for an external management consultant and have continued to be involved in things since then.

Some service users had relevant experience from before they became unwell; others were completely new to this kind of work. A total of 37 users have been involved since the work began. Service user Norman recalls how he first became involved through a session that had been organized to raise staff awareness about mental illness and reduce stigma:

> I agreed to give some information and advice on what I thought they should tell new staff about the experience of mental illness but I did not want to be involved in saying anything myself. But when I realised that they were missing out really important points and not putting it in the right way I could not contain myself and I had to say something. I was enticed to join the people at the front and then we just took off.

Celia explains her motivation to participate:

> My neighbours don't know me except as a person with mental health problems. I didn't like how I was being perceived. I knew I had a hell of a lot to offer and contribute but did not know how to do it.
>
> If I'm feeling very low when I come into a group, by the end, I feel much better and more worthy... I have changed a lot. I'm more interested in what's going on. It has given me strength.

Overcoming initial fears can bring confidence and self-esteem:

> I felt elated after our first presentation, they asked so many questions and I found I knew most of the answers. (Stan, service user)

> On the day of my first presentation, I felt as if I could not even remember my name! Once we started, I enjoyed every moment of it. I recommend the experience to everyone. (Paweł Spocinski, service user)

WHAT DOES THE EDUCATION DEPARTMENT DO?

The Education Department has developed off-the-shelf packages for workshops with schools, colleges and other groups where creative approaches are used to stimulate ideas and discussion. Not only are workshop participants helped to improve their understanding about mental illness by people with personal experience of mental distress but also they are encouraged to consider strategies for improving their own mental health and well-being. Each initiative is created, developed, planned and implemented by the project team with equal involvement of staff, volunteers and service users.

For example the group works with young people aged 14–18 in schools – addressing as many as 200 on one occasion. The team found these students much more knowledgeable and open minded than they had imagined they would be. Unfortunately, it is difficult for teachers to make the additional time that is needed for this vital work.

With a theme of 'Have you ever felt like this?' the team has done sketches using scenarios for school students to discuss. This prompts young people to share feelings and acknowledge their own experiences of anger, anxiety, stress or depression and to talk about how they deal with them and learn about how and where to gain help and support if feelings become overwhelming.

In addition to the contact with schools, users have worked with a major local retailer that offers a buddying scheme to help employees (including those who have had mental health problems) who have been off work for a long time to get back on track. Buddies (i.e. those who were supporting people in the workplace) appeared to have little understanding of mental health issues so, although they wanted to be helpful they did not always know where to start. Jewish Care's mental health awareness training, tailored to meet their needs, gave them the confidence required.

One of the team's major successes was to take their 'chicken soup' initiative to the MIND conference in Harrogate in 2006. Chicken soup is delicious, nourishing and therapeutic – often known as 'Jewish penicillin'. Not only does it have some basic ingredients but also it can be made in many different ways by using a variety of recipes to make it special. This seemed to be a good analogy for user involvement.

Participants in the 'chicken soup' workshop are asked to think in small groups about all the ingredients that are needed for successful user involvement as well as reflecting on the barriers and how these can be overcome. All their suggestions (ingredients) are put into a large chicken soup pot to be shared in the large group. This then forms a creative new recipe for effective user involvement. Service users and staff who participated in this very public event found it exhilarating:

> We created a vibrant atmosphere in debate and discussion. (SU anon)

> After Harrogate I was on a high despite difficulties. We had a wonderful team of ten people sharing quality time together all on an equal par. (Susan, staff member)

The group's most recent project has been to write a two-act play called *Beyond Reason* that explores a young man's experience of psychosis. The team plans to take this out into health trusts, local authorities and other agencies as a trigger to raise awareness. The work of the department is now publicized in a newsletter called *Gesher*, which is edited by the team.

Norman, one of the service users, sums up the key to the project's achievements:

> We have been successful because there has been leadership, encouragement, support and genuine partnership.

CONCLUSION

The problem of stigma in mental health has been clearly articulated by service users, investigated by researchers and denounced by user and carer organizations, professionals and government since the mid-1990s. In spite of hard work, research and campaigning, there has been little impact on the actual lives of people with mental health issues who continue to experience suspicion and rejection. Campaigns have worked best and people with mental distress have benefited most when service users themselves have been actively involved in the activities.

GOOD PRACTICE GUIDANCE FOR CHALLENGING STIGMA

The broader literature and the more local Jewish Care experience indicate the following good practice guidance for challenging stigma:

- Involve service users from the outset.

- Identify the target audience clearly.

- Provide information by drawing on service users' experience.

- Encourage people to acknowledge the mental health issues that they and those close to them also experience.

- Encourage inclusion in employment, leisure, community, sporting and other activities.

- Establish a rigorous system of monitoring impact and evaluate outcomes from service users' perspectives.

REFERENCES

Anthony, W. (1993) 'Recovery from mental illness: the guiding vision of the mental health service system.' *Innovations and Research 2*, 3, 17–25.

BBC News (1999) 'Combating the stigma of mental illness.' *BBC News,* 13 October. Available at http://www.news.bbc.co.uk/1/hi/health/187364.stm, accessed on 12 May 2009.

Beales, A., Beresford, P., Hitchon, G., Westra, A. and Basset, T. (2006) *Service Users Together: A Guide to Involvement.* London: Together.

Branfield, F. and Beresford, P. (2006) *Making User Involvement Work.* York: Joseph Rowntree Foundation.

Callard, F. (2006) *Mind over Matter 2: SHIFT Media Survey Summary Report*. London: Care Services Improvement Partnership. Available at www.kc.csip.org.uk, accessed on 12 May 2009.

Department of Health (1999) *National Service Framework for Mental Health*. London: Department of Health.

Goffman, E. (1968) *Stigma: Notes on the Management of Spoiled Identity*. London: Penguin.

Health Care Commission, Mental Health Act Commission and National Institute for Mental Health in England/Care Services Improvement Partnership (2005) *National Census of Inpatients in Mental Health Hospitals and Facilities in England and Wales*. London: Health Care Commission. Available at www.cqc.org.uk/_db/_ documents/04021746.pdf, accessed on 12 May 2009.

Highland Users' Group (HUG), National Schizophrenia Campaign Scotland, Penumbria, Royal College of Psychiatrists and Scottish Association for Mental Health (2006) *A Review of the First Four Years of the Scottish Anti-Stigma Campaign*. Edinburgh: See Me Scotland. Available at www.seemescotland.org.uk, accessed on 12 May 2009.

Levy, B.R. (2003) 'Mind matters: Cognitive and physical effects of aging self-stereotypes.' *Journals of Geronotology Series B: Psychological Sciences and Social Sciences 58*, 4, 203–211.

Lucas, H., Scammell, A. and Hagelskamp, C. (2005) 'How do GP registrars feel about dealing with mental health issues in the primary care setting? A qualitative investigation.' *Primary Health Care Research and Development 6*, 1, 60–71.

National Institute of Mental Health in England (NIMHE) (2004) *Scoping Review on Mental Health Anti-Stigma and Discrimination: Current Activities and What Works – Executive Summary*. London: NIMHE. Available at www.sesami.org.uk/stigmas coping_summary.pdf, accessed on 12 May 2009.

Office of the Deputy Prime Minister (ODPM) (2004) *Mental Health and Social Exclusion: Social Exclusion Unit Report*. London: ODPM.

Oliver, M. (1990) 'The individual and social models of disability.' Presentation at Joint Workshop of the Living Options Group and the Research Unit of the Royal College of Physicians, 23 July. Available at www.leeds.ac.uk/disability-studies/archiveuk/Oliver/in%20soc%20dis.pdf, accessed on 12 May 2009.

Pembroke, L. (2007) 'We need rights, not another campaign.' *Psychminded*, 2 August. Available at www.psychminded.co.uk/news/news2007/July07/stigma003. htm, accessed on 12 May 2009.

Pilgrim, D. and Rogers, A. (1993) 'Mental health service users' views of medical practitioners.' *Journal of Interprofessional Care 7*, 2, 167–176.

Pinfold, V., Thornicroft, G., Huxley, P. and Farmer, P. (2005) 'Active ingredients in anti-stigma programmes in mental health.' *International Review of Psychiatry 17*, 2, 123–131.

Read, J. and Baker, S. (1996) *Not Just Sticks and Stones: A Survey of the Stigma, Taboos and Discrimination Experienced by People with Mental Health Problems*. London: MIND.

Rethink (2008) 'Nine out of ten people with mental health problems are prisoners of stigma.' London: Rethink. Available at www.politics.co.uk/opinion-formers/

press-releases/rethink-nine-out-ten-people-with-mental-health-problems-are-prisoners-stigma-$1232557$365673.htmm, accessed on 12 May 2009.

Royal College of Psychiatrists (2002) *Changing Minds Campaign (2002–2008).* London: Royal College of Psychiatrists. Available at www.rcpsych.ac.uk/campaigns/changingminds.aspx, accessed on 12 May 2009.

Sartorius, N. and Schulze, H. (2005) *Reducing the Stigma of Mental Illness: A Report from a Global Programme of the World Psychiatric Association.* Cambridge: Cambridge University Press.

Sayce, L. (2000) *From Psychiatric Patient to Citizen.* London: Macmillan.

See Me Anti-Stigma Campaign Scotland (2002) *Users' Voices.* Edinburgh: See Me Scotland. Available at www.seemescotland.org.uk, accessed on 12 May 2009.

Smith, E., Smith, J., Hopps, M. and Lumley, V. (2008) 'Experiencing the Process.' In A. Hall, M. Wren and S. Kirby (eds) *Care Planning in Mental Health: Promoting Recovery.* Oxford: Blackwell.

Stanley, N., Penhale, B., Riordan, D., Barbour, R.S. and Holden, S. (2003) *Child Protection and Mental Health Services.* Bristol: Policy Press.

Taylor, G. and Spencer, S. (2004) *Social Identities: Multidisciplinary Approaches.* Oxford: Routledge.

Thornicroft, G. (2006) *Shunned: Discrimination against People with Mental Illness.* Oxford: Oxford University Press.

Time to Change (2008) *Stigma Shout: Service User Experiences of Stigma and Discrimination.* London: Time to Change, 15–19 The Broadway, London E15 4BQ.

TNS Custom Market Research Company for SHIFT Media Network/Care Services Improvement Partnership (2007) *Attitudes to Mental Illness in England 2007.* London: Department of Health.

Wallcraft, J. (2005) 'Recovery from Mental Breakdown.' In J. Tew (ed.) *Social Perspectives in Mental Health.* London: Jessica Kingsley Publishers.

Wollaston, S. (2008) 'A reality show about mental illness sounds dire – but you might just learn a thing or two.' *Guardian,* 12 November. Available at www.guardian.co.uk/culture/2008/nov/12/lastnight-s-tv-television-bbc, accessed on 12 May 2009.

World Health Organization (2008) *Stigma: An International Briefing Paper.* Edinburgh: NHS Health Scotland.

CHAPTER 9

User Involvement in Planning and Developing Services

Jenny Weinstein with Southwark MIND Council members

INTRODUCTION

> All mental health services must be planned and implemented in partnership with local communities and involve service users and carers. (Department of Health 1999a, p.17)

The government published the above statement with respect to its proposed improvements to mental health services in 1999. The following are some perspectives of a service user (Moreland 2007) about her experience of how these aspirations are working in practice nearly a decade later:

> We are told we cannot attend certain meetings unless we represent a group (most of us are individuals speaking of our own experience now you want us to be at the table on behalf of everyone else who does not or cannot engage)...
>
> ...They should realize that many Service Users do not engage because they are treated badly, made to feel stupid, ignored, condescended to, that is why faces come and go...we get fed up trying to be heard...and in the end we walk away...
>
> ...Yet we are scared to speak up in case our services (if we are lucky enough to have any) are withdrawn.
>
> ...Unless we are truly integrated into the professionals' very existence as part of normal life we will always have a situation of them and us, causing the all too familiar faces of stigma and discrimination from the very people who should know better.

This chapter explores some of the tensions and dilemmas inherent in the conflicting perspectives illustrated by the above quotations. Questions are raised about whether, despite the significant progress that has been made in establishing frameworks for user involvement and the undoubted participation of numerous service users within these frameworks, many people with mental health issues still feel that their voices are not being heard and that the types of services they have been asking for over many decades are still not being developed.

The chapter has been written in partnership with representatives of Southwark MIND, based in inner London, who have shared their experiences of being involved in structures and process for planning and monitoring mental health services in their locality. Southwark MIND is a user-led organization with two paid user employees overseen by a council of elected service users who represent local mental health resources and user groups. The council meets monthly. The first half of its meeting is a closed session and in the second part local mental health managers and service providers are in attendance. This enables the council to raise issues of concern to users in relation to specific services while service providers keep the council updated about proposed changes and developments.

The case studies presented explore participation in a Local Involvement Network (LINk), a partnership board, and a major user-led campaign to improve and retain crisis services. The case studies are contextualized with a brief history of government's responses to users' campaigns for involvement in planning services. The examples given are not intended in any way as a criticism of the local Southwark services or their commitment to user involvement. On the contrary, the authors would argue that the South London and Maudsley NHS Foundation Trust (SLAM) and the London Borough of Southwark are genuinely committed to promoting service user involvement and, moreover, are at the cutting edge of promoting and resourcing this way of working. Rather, the case examples demonstrate that in spite of the tremendous advances in recent years that have been made by progressive trusts such as SLAM in establishing ways of empowering service users to participate, there remain significant cultural, financial and political barriers to be overcome before service users feel they can really make a difference on the important decisions.

BACKGROUND TO USER INVOLVEMENT IN SERVICE PLANNING

As outlined in Chapter 1, mental health service users have been involved in a struggle to influence their conditions since the inmates of what was then known as 'the house of Bedlam' presented their petition to parliament in 1620. An organized movement can be dated from the formation of the Alleged Lunatics' Friends Society in 1845 by former patients to act as a lobbying and campaigning group. The first Patients' Council in Britain was established in Nottingham in 1986 based on models of self-advocacy established in the Netherlands following ill treatment scandals during the 1970s (Van Ginneken 1992). The UK national self-advocacy network Survivors Speak Out was created in the same year. By 1992 more than a hundred local survivor groups had come into being, stimulated by the NHS and Community Care Act 1990 and the introduction of the Mental Illness Specific Grant (MISG) in 1991. These groups became linked up through the creation in 1992 of the United Kingdom Advocacy Network (UKAN).

The rise of service user involvement during the 1970s and 1980s is characterized by Crossley (2002) and Pilgrim (2005) as part of the radical oppositional activity of the period when minority groups such as women, people with disabilities, gays and black people formed loose networks or 'social movements' to fight back against discrimination and oppression. Many campaigning health and social care professionals supported these developments; for example, the ideas of the radical psychiatrist R.D. Laing, who opposed traditional psychiatry (see, for example, Laing 1960), were popular at the time and Cooper (1980) argued that real change can be achieved only with a significant shift in the balance of power by:

- abandoning the humiliating process of a patient being 'interrogated' by a psychiatrist who would then decide on a diagnosis and treatment

- turning the current hierarchy on its head with the mentally ill person driving the agenda and not the doctor

- using a supportive and enabling approach aimed at 'opening up experience' rather than closing it down.

Radical social workers started their own magazine, *Case Con*, to promote user empowerment and undermine what were considered 'oppressive' models of service delivery. The *Case Con Manifesto* (Case Con Collective 1972) states:

> Every day of the week, every week of the year, social workers...see the utter failure of social work to meet the real needs of the people it purports to help...
>
> We are supposed to 'help' our 'clients' by making them 'accept responsibility' – in other words, come to terms as individuals with basically unacceptable situations.

The manifesto goes on to recommend that social workers need to support the people they work with by helping them to take 'collective action' (Case Con Collective 1972).

It was at this period that principles of 'anti-racist', 'anti-sexist' and 'anti-discriminatory practice' became integrated into the value base of social work (Central Council for Education and Training in Social Work 1989) and, in spite of a political backlash in the early 1990s (Pierce and Weinstein 2000), have remained core to social work education and practice ever since. Moreover, following a general acknowledgement of the concept of 'institutional racism and discrimination' (Macpherson 1999), these principles have been introduced into the training and codes of practice of most health and social care professionals, including the police. Even medical education has been influenced, with new doctors being taught to empower patients to manage their own health by offering them 'information' and 'choice' rather than imposing unexplained or mystifying treatments. The concept of the 'expert patient' (Department of Health 2001a) was introduced so that the knowledge and skills of people with experience of particular illnesses or difficulties would be called upon to contribute to the training of professionals (see Chapter 1).

Mental health service users do not have a manifesto as such but the research undertaken to elicit their views about how they would like services to change for example (Pilgrim and Waldron 1999; Rose 2001; Shaping Our Lives National User Network *et al.* 2003) identifies a number of continually recurring themes many of which are summarized by Pilgrim (2005, pp.19–20):

- *The opposition to coercion*, which focuses on the way in which people with mental health problems are stigmatized and segregated from society (see Chapter 8).

- *The opposition to compulsory treatment* – for example evident in the long-running campaigns to ensure that the Mental Health Act

2007 would not jeopardize the rights of people with mental health problems (Mental Health Alliance 2006) and the demands of service users to be involved in decisions about their own care (see Chapter 7).

- *The opposition to psychiatric diagnosis* – as Greaves explains so forcefully in Chapter 3, being labelled is counterproductive in terms of Recovery.

- *The demand for greater treatment choice*, such as access to talking and other alternative therapies, women-only facilities and access to 24-hour non-institutional crisis support.

- *The demand for greater citizenship*, which means social inclusion in employment, leisure, family and social life, illustrated by Greaves in Chapters 3 and 4.

Pilgrim (2005) goes on to argue that:

> User involvement endorses the voice of the patient. It is entreated and attended to, but on terms strictly circumscribed by those controlling the service status quo: managers and professionals. It is in the gift of the latter powerful groups to issue this invitation more or less enthusiastically and with more or less good faith. The existence of mental health services, mental health professionals and their preferred methods of interventions are taken as givens. Professionals and managers may listen to all viewpoints. They may concede feedback and genuinely seek to change services. But they always do so from a position of power. (p.25)

Similar views are expressed in a study that reported the findings of qualitative case studies of user involvement in two mental health provider trusts in London (Rutter *et al.* 2004). Semi-structured interviews were conducted with a variety of stakeholders, including trust staff at all levels and user group members. The researchers found that:

> user involvement remained in the gift of provider managers: providers retained control over decision-making, and expected users to address Trust agendas and conform to Trust management practices. Users wanted to achieve concrete changes to policies and services, but had broader aspirations to improve the status and condition of people with mental health problems. (Rutter *et al.* 2004, p.1973)

An earlier study by Crawford *et al.* (2002) who undertook a qualitative review of 42 papers about the impact of service user involvement, found that although users appreciated being more involved and this aided communication between staff and users, there was no evidence of significant changes in the quality of care received.

For example, the reduction from two types of Care Programme Approach (CPA) – Standard and Enhanced – to only one level is justified by government on the grounds of reducing bureaucracy and providing a more person-centred flexible service to individuals whose condition is not severe (Department of Health 2008a, p.11). It suggests that for people who are stable, formal CPA paperwork is not required but that a plan of care made with the service user should be recorded in a simpler, more flexible format, for example a letter.

However, many service users reported to Southwark MIND that they feared an outcome whereby service users would be treated by services as though they were either 'ill' or 'well' without an acknowledgement of the cyclical nature of many mental health problems and the influence of social or psychological difficulties on mental well-being. They expressed concern that there would be limited support over the transitional period between breakdown and recovery and that no support to prevent further breakdown would be offered. The change was seen as a 'service cut' because, unless there is a formal CPA in operation, there is no obligation on mental health services to provide a care coordinator and a care plan. If a service user was thought to be stable and doing well on their medication, they would be discharged from specialist mental health services back to primary care. MIND's informants believed that these 'stable' service users would remain subject to the same stresses and be vulnerable to a relapse which might be prevented if they continued to have immediate access to specialist mental health services.

It appears that although government policy (Department of Health 1999b, 2006) promotes user-centred services in theory, and mental health service providers are clearly working hard to establish appropriate systems and structures to facilitate this, involvement is often tokenistic and peripheral to the key decisions that continue to be made by the professionals or the budget holders.

STRUCTURES DEVELOPED TO FACILITATE USER INVOLVEMENT IN PLANNING

Community Health Councils (CHCs) were set up by the government in 1974 to monitor and review the National Health Service and to recommend improvements. The CHC was presented as a local independent consumer council for the NHS.

In 2002 the National Health Service Reform and Health Care Professions Act 2002 replaced Community Health Councils in England with a new set of structures headed up by a Commission for Patient and Public Involvement in Health (CPPIH). The aim was to promote the involvement in health of patients and all sections of the community, especially those whose views are not usually heard.

In 2007, the structures were revised yet again by the Local Government and Public Involvement in Health Act 2007. This aimed to strengthen the impact of user involvement by removing any artificial division between health and social care and extending the remit of involvement to include commissioning and scrutiny.

The Local Involvement Networks (Amendment) Regulations (Department of Health 2008b) set out how this should be done by replacing Patient and Public Involvement (PPI) forums with Local Involvement Networks, which would be hosted by an independent voluntary organization (see Chapter 1 for more background to LINks).

The improvements anticipated by government from the new system were that:

- Services may be consulted upon holistically – so that there is no artificial divide between health and social care and no opportunity for providers to abrogate responsibility to the 'other' service.

- The LINks provide an opportunity for regulators to engage with communities and adapt the machinery of regulation.

- The LINks will provide a voice for a wide variety of service users and carers in all services including those whose voices are not often heard, such as young people.

- LINks are being created to help give the whole community the chance to input into the design and delivery of local health and social services by

  ○ creating a positive culture

  ○ aligning organizational structures

  ○ turning information into meaningful evidence

  ○ clarifying roles, rights and responsibilities

  ○ providing tailored training and support

- ○ providing adequate resources

- ○ enabling dialogue and communication

- ○ monitoring, evaluating and disseminating.

The chair of the Commission for Patient and Public Involvement in Health (Grant 2006) expressed some reservations about the new plans, saying that:

- PPI forum members are an asset that we cannot afford to ignore. Their experience and knowledge will be essential in developing and implementing the new system.

- LINks need to be properly resourced, and to have teeth.

- LINks need to be truly independent from the NHS.

LINks are being promoted on the basis of an acknowledgement by government that service users and carers do not always feel they have a strong enough voice to change aspects of their health or social care. A LINks role once it is up and running is to:

- ask people what they think about local health care services and provide a chance to suggest ideas to help improve services

- investigate specific issues of concern to the community

- use its powers to hold services to account and get results

- ask for information and get an answer in a specified amount of time

- be able to carry out spot checks to see if services are working well (carried out under safeguards)

- make reports and recommendations and receive a response

- refer issues to the local 'Overview and Scrutiny Committee'.

(Directgov 2008)

The following case study illustrates some of the challenges being faced to put these excellent objectives into practice.

CASE STUDY 1: LINKS

One of the authors of this chapter was a participant in the initial meeting in her local authority to establish the local LINk. It was very well attended mainly by service users and carers who had been active in the Patient and Public Involvement consultation forums. The meeting itself was run by senior executives from the local authority who, possibly coincidentally, appeared to all be middle-aged white males. The language they used when introducing and conducting the meeting was full of jargon and no attempt was made to communicate in a user-friendly way to meet the needs of (for example) participants with learning disabilities or those whose first language was not English.

A number of concerns were raised by the public about the potential effectiveness of LINks. For example, one service user who had represented patients on her local NHS Trust's patient forum felt that she had been effective because of her close knowledge of the trust and its workings. Her sense was that if the new LINk was to cover all health and social services within the borough, for all service user groups, it would be hard to identify priorities. How would one organization adequately represent the varying interests of say children with disabilities, older people with dementia, mental health service users and older people wanting support to live at home? Would this lead to hierarchies of need and divisions between different user groups?

Worries were also expressed about the genuine independence of the LINk. The local authority had the responsibility for commissioning a local voluntary organization to host the LINk. However, the host had to meet the contract specification set by the local authority and there was concern that this structure could militate against a genuinely user-led organization.

In the author's locality the commissioned voluntary agency facilitated a public meeting of LINk members to elect an interim executive committee. These individuals, all of whom were unpaid volunteers, had had previous experience in the various structures described above. Some representatives had been involved in NHS patient forums, some were part of disability groups, some were from ethnic minority lobby groups and others were from groups that linked with social services. There were no mental health service users or carers on the executive. This diverse group of individuals was told that their brief would be to coordinate user participation and consultation across all of health and social care in their area. In order to help them deal with this extensive brief, a one-day training course was being organized for them.

Local critics of the approach have complained that:

- All communication about the LINk has been via email, thus excluding service users who do not have access to the internet.

- Many key groups are not represented, such as people with mental health problems or learning disabilities.

- The complexity of the brief means that executive members, who are not professionals but service users who have had experience of advocating within familiar settings and services, are having to struggle with lengthy documents covering aspects of services about which they have minimal knowledge.

- The excellent role these individuals were playing in their own services has now been lost.

Not surprisingly, when the time came for elections for a permanent executive, many of the interim executive resigned because they felt out of their depth. They were replaced by two prospective parliamentary candidates, two ex-councillors, one prospective councillor, and three retired social services managers who took most of the lead roles, working with a small rump of original interim executive members. This new group was then wooed by the health and social care providers and invited to sit on all sorts of consultative groups. The concern was that by involving these individuals who were members of LINks, the providers might feel able to tick boxes to say they had consulted with user and patient representatives.

Clearly this is only one case example from one locality and it is early days at the time of writing. Nevertheless, it may be challenging for this new centralized structure, consisting entirely of volunteers, to increase participation and control by service users in the everyday planning, quality assurance and running of services.

CASE STUDY 2: LOCAL PARTNERSHIP BOARDS

Partnership Boards are non-statutory bodies that offer the opportunity to create a forum that brings statutory and non-statutory representatives together with user, carer and provider groups in order to improve the experience of needs assessment, planning, delivery and service performance (Community Services Improvement Partnership 2006). The boards were introduced in *Valuing People: A New Strategy for Learning Disability for the*

21st Century (Department of Health 2001b) with a remit for 'overseeing the interagency planning and commissioning of comprehensive, integrated and inclusive services that provide a genuine choice of service options to people in the local community' (p.106). The boards have now been extended to cover any care group or service-led approach, for example Older People Services and Mental Health Services.

SLAM was one of the first Mental Health Trusts to establish local Partnership Boards in each of the local authorities that it served. The board consists of all the stakeholders from the relevant NHS and social services agencies, as well as voluntary agencies who have an interest in mental health commissioning and service delivery. Southwark MIND Council, which entirely comprises mental health service users, sends two of its members to the Southwark Partnership Board to represent mental health service users.

The Partnership Board develops and monitors local implementation targets that have been agreed as part of SLAM's overall strategic plan, following consultation with all stakeholders. The service user agenda to influence planning and implementation is that the strategy must:

- be recovery orientated – promoting self-actualization

- ensure that 'Recovery' is not being interpreted simply as 'getting people back to work'

- ensure that all service users are able to define what Recovery means to them

- ensure that all interventions are person-centred

- not give all the power of decision-making to psychiatrists

- encourage service user run services and reduce institutionalization

- facilitate peer advocacy by service users.

This reflects the requirements identified in a wider consultation with service users about what they wanted from services (Commission for Social Care Inspection 2006) which included:

- choice

- flexibility

- accessible accurate information

- being treated with respect

- being allowed to take risks

- fairness and non-discrimination

- support to be safe.

Examples of how some of these principles operate in SLAM are a project to reduce occupancy in high security forensic settings and enable people to live in the community with much stronger support networks and a user-focused monitoring project (Bertram 2002) known as the South London User Research Project (SLURP) to identify what service users and carers want from their local services.

Southwark MIND values its representation on the Partnership Board because it is very helpful to be part of the discussions and to feed back information about developments to the other users on the council and express their views at the board. Nevertheless, user representatives can have only a limited impact on major decisions about the planning and development of services. MIND Council takes the view that service users will be able to have a really meaningful influence only when they can be fully involved in the tendering process. This would mean drawing up the specifications for the service required, shortlisting the tenders received and being on the selection panel. Users would then need to have some input into the service level agreement and the contract and to be play a key role in monitoring and audit of the performance of the contractor.

Changing the culture takes time, especially when such fundamental shifts in decision-making processes are required. In recognition of concerns expressed by users that their involvement is still tokenistic to some extent, a steering group has been established to further progress the SLAM model of service user and carer involvement.

CASE STUDY 3: CAMPAIGN TO SAVE THE MAUDSLEY EMERGENCY CLINIC

In relating this case study it is important to acknowledge that the story is told from the perspective of the service users. It does not purport to be a balanced account – offering the service provider's viewpoint – because the purpose of the case study is to illustrate both the strengths and the limitations of a user-led campaign. The story is related by two members of Southwark MIND Council who were active and involved throughout the campaign.

In 2004 it became clear that the Maudsley Emergency Clinic was being considered for closure. Service users became very upset because this is one of the only services where users have direct 24-hour access to mental health services without the need for referral and this is something that they value. The clinic had given people a place of safety and security. It was regarded as an accessible haven where they felt known and understood.

SLAM, which ran the service, convened an Emergency Services Review Group. The remit of this group was to take a wider perspective on emergency services within the Trust and the role of the Emergency Clinic within these. The review group included six service users, representatives from police, Accident and Emergency, Southwark Social Services Department, SLAM and other relevant organizations. This group organized a stakeholder consultation event to determine what people wanted from crisis services, what aspects needed to be safeguarded and what new services are required.

A management consultant was taken on to consider different proposals for different configurations. Primary care services, the Community Mental Health Team (CMHT), Home Treatment Services and Accident and Emergency services were all consulted. The idea was to draw up a number of different proposals for consultation from which a preferred option would be identified.

The local users' network is very strong and news went round quickly. This led to the establishment of the Lambeth and Southwark Users' Campaign Group, who were very active in lobbying their respective councils and making representations to SLAM. The media picked this up and there was a good coverage in local and even national newspapers.

As part of their campaign, the service users offered to develop their own option to which the Primary Care Trusts (PCTs) and SLAM agreed. The service users wanted a social model with counselling available – not a medical or hospital orientated model. They wanted this to be offered at the Maudsley Hospital, because this is a world-renowned mental health resource familiar to users where many of them were well known. The users were very disappointed when they were told that their option was too expensive. When the draft consultative paper came out with the range of options, the proposal put forward by the service users had been withdrawn.

MIND organized its own stakeholder consultation meeting and found support for saving the Emergency Clinic from people on the ground. The police liked the unit; mainstream Accident and Emergency staff did not feel appropriately equipped to deal with mental health emergencies; staff at the clinic did not want it to close. From the user perspective, one of their key principles for a crisis service was that they could self-refer. Some of the proposals for an out-of-hours crisis service involved having to find a health or care professional who would agree to make a referral.

There followed a well-orchestrated service-user-led campaign that included a demonstration against cuts in mental health services, features on the BBC London website, sustained press publicity, petitions to the local Members of Parliament, who faced questions on the doorstep when they were electioneering, and a debate in the House of Commons. Issues were raised at the local PPI forums and the campaign featured in arts-orientated events such as the Bonkers Festival (an event that celebrates the creativity of people with mental health issues) and produced striking posters and flyers.

Because of the level of opposition in the community, the clinic could not be closed prior to scrutiny of proposals by the secretary of state. This was a significant victory for service users, who felt that they had had some genuine influence through their campaigning. Inevitably, the secretary of state supported the closure but committed an additional £15 million to improve mental health services at the nearby King's College Hospital, which would provide specialist mental health emergency services. The determination of service users to continue their opposition was such that in response to the minister's decision, they decided to seek legal advice. They wanted to know whether, having introduced legislation stating that significant changes cannot be made without consultation with local people, whether the government could then ignore the views expressed through that consultation process. It seemed that by consulting the public and users about their alternative plans, the government was within the law.

Despite service users making persuasive representation at the meetings, Southwark and Lambeth PCTs rubber-stamped the closure of the Emergency Clinic, simply adding that 'we note users have concerns'. Promises were made that services will be monitored carefully and users would remain involved. A group to monitor Crisis Services was established and is being managed by Southwark MIND Executive. This group will continue to undertake public consultation, using focus groups, to ensure that the new arrangements to be put in place – 'a safe segregated area for mental health service users' within King's College Hospital Accident and Emergency – are fit for purpose.

CONCLUSION

There is no doubt that significant efforts are being made by most health and social services organizations to involve service users in the planning and development of services. The government has made its commitment clear by writing a requirement for local consultation into legislation and for requiring clear local structures to facilitate full participation by users in joined up health and care provision. Although the case studies presented here clearly illustrate the progress that has been made by providers in this respect, they also demonstrate how complex the problems are and how many barriers – professional and managerial cultures, financial decision-making and their bureaucracy – impede the processes from bringing about the fundamental changes that service users have been seeking for decades. While service users appreciate the significant improvements in trying to involve them since the government's Patient and Public Involvement initiative in 2003, they still feel that it is sometimes 'empty rhetoric' with policy being made on the basis of sound bites that do not result in any real change in the service user experience on the ground.

GOOD PRACTICE GUIDANCE FOR INVOLVING SERVICE USERS

- Ensure that the time, length and venue of meetings involving users take their comfort and support needs into account.

- Make appropriate transport available to service users who require it.

- Provide refreshments, ensuring that dietary and cultural needs are taken into account.

- Brief and de-brief users so that they fully understand the content and process of the meeting/activity.

- Provide documents in an easy-to-read format and avoid jargon.

- Involve service users from the outset; do not wait until the agenda, strategy or outline plans are already fixed.

REFERENCES

Bertram, M. (2002) 'User involvement and mental health: Critical reflections on critical issues.' Psychminded, 15 December. Available at www.psychminded. co.uk/news/news2002/1202/User%20Involvement%20and%20mental%20 health%20reflections%20on%20critical%20issues.htm, accessed on 12 May 2009.

Case Con Collective (1972) *The Case Con Manifesto.* Available at www.radical.org. uk/barefoot/casecon.htm, accessed on 12 May 2009.

Central Council for Education and Training in Social Work (CCETSW) (1989) *Rules and Requirements for the Diploma in Social Work.* (CCETSW) Paper 30. London: CCETSW.

Commission for Social Care Inspection (2006) *Real Voices, Real Choices: The Qualities People Expect from Care Services.* London: Community Services Improvement Partnership. Available at www.nihme.csip.org.uk/silo/files/csci-real-choices-real-voices.pdf, accessed on 12 May 2009.

Community Services Improvement Partnership (CSIP) (2006) *Partnership Boards.* London: Community Services Improvement Partnership. Available at ww.networks.csip.org.uk, accessed on 10 October 2008.

Cooper, D. (1980) *The Language of Madness.* Harmondsworth: Pelican.

Crawford, M.J., Rutter, D., Manley, C., Weaver, T. *et al.* (2002) 'Systematic review of involving patients in the planning and development of health care.' *British Medical Journal 325*, 7375, 1263.

Crossley, N. (2002) 'Mental health, resistance and social movements: The collective-confrontational dimension.' *Health Education Journal 61*, 2, 138–52.

Department of Health (1999a) *Modern Standards and Service Models: Mental Health.* London: Department of Health.

Department of Health (1999b) *Of Primary Importance: Inspection of Social Services Departments' Links with Primary Care Groups. Working in Partnership: Joint Working between Health and Social Services in Primary Care Groups.* London: Department of Health.

Department of Health (2001a) *The Expert Patient: A New Approach to Chronic Disease Management for the 21st Century.* London: Department of Health.

Department of Health (2001b) *Valuing People: A New Strategy for Learning Disability for the 21st Century*, Cm 5086. London: The Stationery Office.

Department of Health (2006) *Our Health, Our Care, Our Say: A New Direction for Community Services*, Cm 6737. London: The Stationery Office.

Department of Health (2008a) *Refocusing the Care Programme Approach.* London: Department of Health.

Department of Health (2008b) *The Local Involvement Networks (Amendment) Regulations Statutory Instruments No.1877.* London: Department of Health. Available at www. opsi.gov.uk/si/si2008/uksi_20081877_en_1, accessed on 12 May 2009.

Directgov (2008) *Health and Social Care Local Involvement Networks (LINks).* London: Directgov. Available at www.direct.gov.uk/en/HealthAndWellBeing/Health-Services/PractitionersAndServices/DG_071867, accessed on 12 May 2009.

Grant, S. (2006) 'Commission for Patient and Public Involvement in Health comments on new Local Involvement Networks.' London: NHS Networks. Available at www.networks.nhs.uk/news.php?nid=911, accessed on 12 May 2009.

HM Government (2002) *National Health Service Reform and Health Care Professions Act 2002.* London. The Stationery Office.

HM Government (2007) *Local Government and Public Involvement in Health Act.* London: The Stationery Office.

Laing, R.D. (1960) *The Divided Self.* London: Penguin.

Macpherson, W. (1999) *The Stephen Lawrence Inquiry,* Cm 4262–1 London: The Stationery Office. Available at www.archive.official-documents.co.uk/document/cm42/4262/4262.htm, accessed on 12 May 2009.

Mental Health Alliance (2006) 'Updated Mental Health Act must be fit for twenty first century says alliance,' 23 March. London: Mental Health Alliance. Available at www.mentalhealthalliance.org.uk/news/amended83act.html, accessed on 12 May 2009.

Moreland, M. (2007) *Mental Health Service User Movement?* BBC action network site. Available at www.bbc.co.uk/dna/collective/A19232705, accessed on 12 May 2009.

Pierce, R. and Weinstein, J. (2000) *Innovative Education and Training for Care Professionals.* London: Jessica Kingsley Publishers.

Pilgrim, D. (2005) 'Protest and Co-option.' In A. Bell and P. Lindley (eds) *Beyond the Water Towers: The Unfinished Revolution in Mental Health Services 1986–2005.* London: Sainsbury Centre for Mental Health.

Pilgrim, D. and Waldron, L. (1999) 'User involvement in mental health service development: How far can it go?' *Journal of Mental Health 7,* 1, 95–104.

Rose, D. (2001) *Users' Voices: The Perspectives of Mental Health Service Users on Community and Hospital Care.* London: Sainsbury Centre for Mental Health.

Rutter, D., Manley, C., Weaver, T., Crawford, M.J. and Fulop, N. (2004) 'Patients or partners? Case studies of user involvement in the planning and delivery of adult mental health services in London.' *Social Science and Medicine 58,* 10, 1973–1984.

Shaping Our Lives National User Network, Black User Group (West London), Footprints and Waltham Forest Black Service User Group, and Service Users' Action Forum (Wakefield) (2003) *Shaping Our Lives: What People Think of the Social Care Services They Use.* York: Joseph Rowntree Foundation.

Van Ginneken, P. (1992) '10 Years of Patient Advocacy in the Netherlands.' In J. Casselman, D. Bobon, P. Cosyns, J. Wilmotte *et al.* (eds) *Law and Mental Health.* London: Sage.

CHAPTER 10

User Involvement in Research

Tony Leiba

INTRODUCTION AND BACKGROUND

Service users of health and social care have the experience and skills to complement those of researchers. They know what it feels like to undergo treatments and their various side-effects; they have ideas about what questions should be asked and how questions may be asked differently. Furthermore, if the needs and views of users are reflected in research, results are more likely to be obtained which can be used to improve health and social care practice.

This chapter will present and examine service user involvement and user-controlled research in health and social care, emphasizing the benefits and the challenges, then go on to draw on the experiences of users and a researcher in a collaborative research project.

The Department of Health (1998, 1999, 2000), Consumers in NHS Research Support Unit (1999), research charities (Joseph Rowntree Foundation 2005) and funding bodies have all emphasized the importance of user involvement in research. Useful briefing notes have been produced, and there is information about how the process works in practice, and the philosophical, conceptual, confidentiality, ethical and practical challenges that may arise for researchers and service users. The massive imbalance of power that exists in services between professionals, researchers and users makes working together particularly challenging (Lindow 2001).

Research now has a high profile and there is emphasis on the importance of evidence. As a result national organizations were established to help provide the knowledge base for health and social care provision;

for instance, the National Institute for Health and Clinical Excellence (NICE), the Social Care Institute for Excellence (SCIE) and the National Institute for Mental Health for England (NIMHE), subsequently integrated into the Care Services Improvement Partnership (CSIP). At the same time there has been a massive expansion of the interest in user involvement in research and evaluation. This growing interest demonstrates an unwillingness to be deferential to research and researchers and an increasing sense that service users have a right to have a say in research and to critically evaluate research (Beresford 2003).

User involvement in research embraces user-led, collaborative and participatory research activities. These different approaches tend to employ a qualitative methodology, with a minority of service user researchers engaging in the quantitative paradigm. It would be of value to service users and to researchers, to develop more participatory and emancipatory quantitative research activities, which employ the humanistic qualities of qualitative research. In so doing user involvement may help to break down the traditional notion of what is good and worthwhile research. The helpful comparisons between Tilakaratna's (1990) definitions of 'elitist' research and 'participatory research' are outlined below.

TRADITIONAL (ELITIST) RESEARCH

Tilakaratna (1990, p.1) suggests that in elitist research 'the fundamental assumption is that "ordinary" people are incapable of doing research – it is a monopoly of the elite who know scientific methodologies.' Ordinary people can only be the subjects of research who are observed or questioned in surveys and questionnaires to provide material for 'experts' to analyse without any input from the people from whom data was collected. The outcome is written up, often in inaccessible jargon or academic language, which only a limited group of individuals will access or understand. 'The people who have been researched are in general not the beneficiaries of this process. The knowledge is not returned to the people' (Tilakaratna (1990, p.2). Without the input of the research subjects, it is suggested, the findings may be hard to apply because they 'fail to capture the perceptions of the people and their living realities' (Tilakaratna 1990, p.2).

USER-LED RESEARCH

User-led research involves service users controlling all stages of the research process, obtaining funding, design, recruitment, data collection, data analysis, writing the report and dissemination. An example of a user-led initiative is the Service User Research Enterprise (SURE), which undertakes research that tests the effectiveness of services and treatments from the perspective of people with mental health problems and their carers. SURE was launched in 2000 at the Institute of Psychiatry, King's College London. SURE has a co-director who is a service user researcher and the first senior lecturer in user-led research in Europe (Rose 2003). SURE's first national study, Patients' Perspectives on Electroconvulsive Therapy (ECT) (Rose, Wykes and Leese 2004), was a Department of Health commissioned systematic review of what patients thought about electroconvulsive therapy. The results influenced the NICE guidance about obtaining consent to ECT and giving information about the treatment. An analysis of research papers, reports by user organizations and first-hand testimonies from service users showed that about half the people receiving the treatment felt that they had not received enough information about the procedure and its common side-effect of memory loss. About one-third felt that they had not freely consented, as they must do by law, even when they had signed a consent form. Two of the researchers in this project had received ECT themselves. SURE's research projects have continued to centre on issues important to service users. They undertake studies relevant to the priorities of service users and carers and they employ people with experience of using mental health services to build both the capacity of the unit and to increase the number of service user researchers.

COLLABORATIVE RESEARCH

Collaborative research tries to weave features of user-led research into large research projects with the service users' role being to carry out the user-led component. With collaborative research power differentials are compounded. Even if a service user researcher has all the requisite degrees, they are unlikely to have the same career track record as general research staff. Service users are more likely to have interruptions in their careers due to illness. There is still stigma, discrimination and being seen as somebody's patient that prevent people who have experienced mental illness from being selected for research posts. Service users are usually seen as junior and they may not receive a salary at all; if they do receive one, it might be therapeutic earnings despite their substantial input (Rose 2003).

PARTICIPATORY RESEARCH

Participatory or action research (Stringer 2004) has emerged as a significant methodology for intervention, development and change within communities and groups. Therefore it is popular with user-involved, user-led and collaborative research projects. Participatory research seeks to reduce elitism and demystify research, thereby making it an intellectual tool which everyone can use to improve their lives. In sharp contrast to elitist research, participatory research is a praxis rhythm of action and reflection where knowledge creation supports action; there is a built-in mechanism to ensure authenticity and genuineness of the information that is generated because people themselves use the information for life improvement. The key features identified by Tilakaratna (1990, p.2) include the following:

- People are both the researchers and the respondents.

- The dichotomy between subject and object is broken.

- People themselves collect the data, and then process and analyse the information using methods easily understood by them.

- The knowledge generated is used to promote actions for change or to improve existing local actions or interventions in care and treatment.

- The knowledge belongs to the people and they are the primary beneficiaries of the knowledge creation.

- Research and action are inseparable, they represent a unity.

Intrinsically the political nature of participation is empowerment and empowerment is both personal and political. On a personal level it builds capacity and confidence and on a political level it enables service users to influence policy and service developments. Participatory approaches to research and inquiry into health and social care by service users rest on the right service users have to put forward their own realities; the particular expertise they have in doing so, which gives added value; and the opportunities it can give them to influence policy and practice.

Participatory forms of research and inquiry are unlikely in themselves to achieve social change, but they can be used by existing organizations to strengthen their own voice, and they can help create new relationships for bringing about change in the longer term.

ETHICAL ISSUES

All research investigations taking place within the NHS or elsewhere must be approved by the responsible ethical committee. Such ethical committees address the issues of beneficence, which is that the research is for the common good and non-maleficence, which is that the research should do no harm. These principles are to protect service users. The paperwork for ethical committee consent is often more suitable for drug trials, than for a collaborative and participatory investigation, and there are still not enough ethical committees with user representatives who talk from the perspective of service users.

The ethical issues are the same whatever the research. However, with user-involved research, it is important to discuss with the people taking part what the limits are during the consent process. There must also be procedures for support arrangements for all the participants in the research. The issues of ending the research must be sensitively handled and the end point must be made clear at the beginning. Lindow (2002) argued that control of the ending processes can be considered as an aspect of power which the researcher has over the researched, therefore, in all user-involved research, all aspects of power relations must be transparent. Researching with other service users brings to the situation the issue of self-disclosure. It is important that people know that they are being studied by their peers, and the researchers need to develop procedures and policies about confidentiality and about how disclosure takes place and how far it might go. Finally, the plans for feedback to the participants and the wider dissemination and publication must be thoughtfully dealt with.

User involvement in research is challenging and it should not be regarded as an add-on to existing research approaches and strategies. It raises fundamental issues, both ideological and ethical, which have far reaching implications for what is understood by research governance and indeed research itself.

THE PROCESSES OF EFFECTIVE USER INVOLVEMENT IN RESEARCH

Drawing mainly from work done in mental health by Hanley (2003), the Mental Health Research Network (2005) and Royle *et al.* (2001) guidance, comments and information are provided to researchers and service users who wish to develop collaborative and participatory research projects.

The degree of service user involvement can be subdivided into four categories. First is researcher-initiated collaboration where service users are consulted but do not share power in the decision-making. Second is user involvement where users play a role in the various research activities but all the control remains with the researcher(s). Third is a true joint collaboration or partnership, which involves an active ongoing partnership between service users and researchers in all the research process from proposal to dissemination. Fourth is a service user initiated and led research project where service users are fully in control because they themselves design, undertake and disseminate the results of a research project.

BENEFITS OF INVOLVEMENT

The user perspective brings with it insights into what it feels like to experience mental health problems, to use mental health services or to receive treatments. Furthermore, service users can help to ensure that the content of the research is more relevant to clinical practice and the results more relevant to them (Hanley 2003). Wykes (2003) develops the argument further by stating three areas where user involvement may change clinical research for the better: improving scientific quality through changing the research questions for the better; changing the outcome measures, by making them more related to the ones that are important to service users; and by amending the method of the research, for example ensuring the randomized control trial approach includes the views of service users. Ramon (2000) argues that user involvement leads to the generation of new and more in-depth knowledge, more truthful information from the research participants, and a better understanding by researchers of the lives of service users.

EARLY INVOLVEMENT

It is vital to ensure that service users can be involved in early discussions about the research, because if this does not happen, many decisions about the research may already have been made without the involvement of service users thereby reducing their potential to influence the research project. Rose (2003) emphasizes the importance of building relationships and capacity for the future by being in touch with users long before a research project starts, offering training and opportunities to enable service users to achieve relevant research qualifications if they want to, or to be trained as interviewers and facilitators of focus groups. All these initiatives seek to avoid the tokenism of inviting one or two service users onto a research advisory group at the last minute, when a research project has already been established, designed and funded.

Furthermore, researchers must ensure that they take account of the diversity of the population. When looking at capacity building, researchers must include people from ethnic minority communities as well as people with different mental illness diagnosis, taking into account issues relating to gender, sexuality and physical disabilities.

POWER AND NEGOTIATION

Trivedi and Wykes (2002) argue that negotiation between researchers and service uses may be one of the most challenging aspects of user involvement, because working in collaboration or partnership usually involves a shift of power from professionals to lay people which some professionals may find hard to deal with. They advocate formalizing the collaboration or partnership with an explicit agreement about how they will work together, including such issues as how service users will be involved, payment and acknowledgement of service users' contributions and facilitating clarity, transparency and flexibility. The power of language must not be overlooked so the use of a jargon-free language is necessary to prevent the resentment felt by service users who feel excluded by the use of inaccessible language and academic research jargon.

Consultations may be a single one with a group of service users, or may involve regular meetings or an invitation to service users to join an existing research group or meeting. Ensure that the service users receive adequate information about the nature of the consultation meeting well in advance. Always involve more than one service user in any advisory group, consultation or meeting, whether it is a one-off meeting or a group meeting regularly over a period of time. Where service users are in a minority in a group or meeting, ensure that the chair is well briefed to enable the group to hear from the service user members. The language used in written material and in the meetings must be jargon free and be fully explained. Refreshment and suitable breaks along with payment must be provided.

Collaboration or partnership occur when service users are involved from the very inception of a research project if they are to have real influence over the direction of the project and the way in which it is to be carried out. At the design stage, ensure that a full assessment is made of the required resources in terms of both time and money. Flexibility should be built in from the beginning to address issues such as the capacity to reschedule the timetable or to provide for extra time if needed. Researchers and service users need to find ways of dealing with distress if and when it arises. For example, service users may need a mentor or someone to contact should they become unwell. Researchers and research managers need to assess whether service users will need an honorary contract. Usually the research governance within the NHS requires all researchers not employed by the NHS to hold an honorary contract if they are to interact with individuals in a way that has a direct bearing on the health care they receive.

TRAINING

The value of research training for service users and researchers is of utmost importance. For service users it is the means of gaining the necessary research skills and should include aspects such as developing proposals, methodologies, data analysis, report writing and dissemination. For service users and researchers, training should be provided jointly in how to work effectively in collaboration, to help to break down the barriers on either side. Townsend and Braithwaite (2002) argued that training provides service users with skills for the immediate project and for the future, thus giving people the confidence to participate, and the opportunity for mutual support. Lockey et al. (2004) offered some suggestions for training provision:

- Training must have a clear aim and purpose, address specific research tasks and real research problems, and draw on the participants' experiences.

- A supportive teaching and learning environment should be created using exercises, small group work and role play.

- Participants must feel confident to challenge in a safe environment.

- Considerable time and space are required to allow all participants to make a full contribution.

- Attention must be paid to the challenge of language because all the stakeholders need to understand each others' language.

SUPPORT

Allam *et al.* (2004) argued that support should be available at every step of the research journey, and that there should be systems within the research environment to prevent undue stress being placed on the service user. Support can be subdivided into practical support for administration and expenses, support through mentorship, supervision and debriefing, and emotional support for example, peer support, and time to talk through difficulties. Providing support does not mean acting as clinician, it is important that researchers and research supervisors do not act as clinicians to service user researchers. Support is essential when differences of opinion occur, because the way in which this is dealt with and resolved will require respect on both sides to ensure that users' views are taken into account in such situations.

The next section provides a practice example of user involvement in research. It is offered here in an honest account to demonstrate both the strengths and the challenges involved in collaborative research projects. The title of the research project was: *Users' views of their care during and after crisis situations/incidents. How should such crisis situations/incidents be prevented, managed and resolved?* A full reference is not provided because this is not in the public domain and in order to maintain the confidentiality of the users and the trust.

USER AND RESEARCHER EXPERIENCES IN A COLLABORATIVE RESEARCH PROJECT

Setting up the project

The research project aimed to capture the views of users about their care and treatment when they were in crisis and admitted to a trust facility, by asking users to reflect on and examine constructively the treatment and care they had received, and to state how they would have wanted to be treated and cared for. The research project was jointly designed and developed with users so as to achieve findings which reflected the users' views rather than those of health and social care professionals.

It was intended that the findings would inform staff about their caring and therapeutic skills before, during and after perceived user crises; provide staff with insights into how they were seen by users; inform staff on how users would have liked to be cared for and treated; point out to staff the effective therapeutic skills which existed and were experienced; identify the areas of care and therapeutic skills which could be considered for improving services and inform practice through education and training.

The methodology resided within the realms of qualitative participatory research, with users being involved from steering group membership, through to the planning, designing, proposal writing, ethical and funding application, all the research activities associated with information collection, analysis, critical reading of the report and dissemination.

The interviewers and interviewees were the users, and the researcher supported the interviewing. The research population was drawn from users who were in acute care during the previous six months and aged between 18 and 65 years of age, both men and women; 25 users came forward as informants. The methods used were one-to-one interviews and the writing of documents or stories in response to questions provided by an interview schedule. Funding was provided by the trust and the research project took two years to complete. The issues highlighted by this research collaboration were warmth in the interactions, cooperation and some challenges.

The consultation process was greeted with enthusiasm, because the agenda was not already set, and the users realized that they would have the major say in what the research should be. This took about three months to set up and process because there was a need to build up the collaborative relationship. This time was needed to build up trust and expertise, and provided for the different working practices, family needs, therapy sessions, social commitments and mental health needs of service users, which may have affected their attendance. The area to be researched was decided on after many meetings and discussions, but finally the title was decided on because it was of intrinsic interest to the service users as well as to the researcher.

Working in partnership with others asks for everyone to have their say and to be able to influence the course of events. What is sometimes insufficiently acknowledged, however, is that there may be disagreements and tensions between the research partners as well as agreements and productive collaboration. The word partnership implies that all the participants get along, but of course that is not necessarily the case. During this research project the difficult relationships took up lots of time and energy, and led to frustration with the work which resulted in some un-comfortable compromises. For example, questions were asked of the re-searcher about why was user involvement sought, and of service users about why they were taking part; the discussions were uncomfortable at times as expectations, clarity, transparency and roles were debated and decided on. Users reminded the researcher that they sometimes have anx-ieties and fears about discussions in the large group, so time and space must be made available for one-to-one conversations with the researcher. The ethics committee members were suspicious about the employment of service user researchers and the methodology, so needed assurance about training, support and levels of risk. Training (see Lockey *et al.* 2004) was provided by the researcher and experienced users on interviewing and note-taking. The challenges related to time, venue and attendance and there was a need to be flexible and accessible throughout the train-ing programme. Users wanted to know if the training could be linked to academic credits such as national vocational qualifications, or with a further education college or a university. This was not a part of the plans for this research, but provided a learning point that when planning user research training it is wise to achieve academic accreditation for such training courses.

Nevertheless, the training had enormous value for the participants' personal development and confidence. Users found different aspects of the research process more difficult than expected, therefore support had to be made available at every step of the journey. Users said that travel-ling to and from unfamiliar places to meet people whom they have not met before proved to be stressful, particularly at dusk; they also felt that interviewers should work in pairs. The users were critical of the content of the training; they said that any research training skills must include active listening and how to manage emotions in the interview situation, because it was difficult to know how to respond when an interviewee became tearful or emotional.

There is a need to pay people appropriately for their contribution to research, whether as research assistants or as informants. For this re-search project the funding provided for only a small fee to be paid to the informants and interviewees and travelling expenses for the interviewers and research assistants. This was insufficient and there were heated dis-cussions that brought strength of feelings about payment of service users undertaking or participating in research. It was felt by the service users that a realistic payment goes some way towards balancing the power dif-ferentials between researchers and service users, and acknowledging the real contribution being made to the project. There are, however, barriers to realistic payments. Users who are in receipt of benefits face a number of limitations on the payments they can receive. The users stated that their payments should be similar to that of the researcher, and that they should receive travel and subsistence expenses for training and for child care or the provision of crèche facilities.

Findings and dissemination of the research

This research project aimed to capture the views of users about their care and treatment when they were in crisis and admitted to a trust facility, and the following were the major findings and recommendations:

- Staff provided users with prescribed medications, plus other social, group and psychotherapeutic interventions.

- Users felt that their medications were poorly explained with insufficient information and in some instances they received explanations only at a later date.

- Users required staff to listen to them and to spend time with them.

- Staff needed to be more sensitive to service users and enable them to participate more fully in their care.

- Staff needed to listen to the service users' own explanation of their situations.

- Staff need to improve their interpersonal relations with service users.

- Care and treatment by other therapists require a higher profile because treatment should be more than just drugs.

- Service users need more information about how to go about complaining about staff's behaviour towards them.

For service users, there was little to be gained from taking part in the research if the findings were not going to be published or used in some way to inform the trust. They were all motivated to help to write the report and to engage in conferences and publications. However, those dissemination activities did not happen as planned. The researcher ended up writing the first draft of the report and two service users acted as critical readers. The final report was circulated to the users who participated, to the user group that worked with the research project and to the trust. Two users and the researcher presented the research findings to the trust's research and development conference.

CONCLUSION

Service users are not a homogenous group; they represent a rich diversity of people in society, whether defined by age, race, ethnicity, religion, disability, gender or sexuality. Service user involvement in research is increasingly gaining recognition as being central to health and social care policy and practice.

The research project described in this chapter was enjoyable, rewarding and demanding. The time and effort put in by service users was significant despite their other commitments, barriers to attending or problems with their mental health. Working with service users made a difference to the research process because it grounded the whole project in the real lived experience of people living with mental health problems.

For many service users, there is little point in carrying out research without the intention of implementing the findings. Some users' main motivation for becoming involved in research may well be a commitment to changing and improving services. This presents a challenge in circumstances where researchers do not have the power to implement the findings and recommendations of their own research. It is therefore important to be clear about any limitations and to address this issue at the outset.

Involving service users in research and supporting user-led research is both challenging and also profitable, not only for users, carer and researchers, but also for the health and social care services generally. If user led, user focused, collaborative and participatory research does become part of the mainstream, this will likely provide some new forms of evidence upon which to base practice. Users come to the research endeavour with a different perspective from that of professionals and are able to elucidate how services and treatments feel to service users, from the inside. They can provide fresh insights, and so research done from this perspective should lead to services that are more acceptable to consumers than many find them today.

GOOD PRACTICE GUIDANCE FOR USER INVOLVEMENT IN RESEARCH

- When inviting users to be involved, it is necessary to ensure that the diversity of the population is taken into account as well as people with different mental illness diagnosis.

- Service users must be involved from the start of a research project.

- Always involve more than one service user in any advisory or steering group meeting.

- Ensure that the provision of support for service users is included in the plans. Adequate support is vital, and it must be practical and educational, and attend to emotional feelings and research-related issues.

- Clarity and transparency is required from the start, about the nature, aims and hoped-for outcomes of the research project.

- Researchers must use plain language and avoid unnecessary jargon.

- Consult with service users with integrity, trust and respect about how their views will be taken on board.

- It is helpful to establish a contract outlining roles, rights and responsibilities of all parties.

- Researchers must be clear about payment, training and the supervision to be provided.

- Training in the relevant knowledge and skills is vital for both service users and researchers.

- Flexibility needs to be built into the research programme; this has implications for funders and commissioners of research to allow greater flexibility in timescales and resources.

- Some resources must be set aside for external and or peer support.

- Good communication with the finance department needs to take place at an early stage, so that the project can have cash available when it is needed.

- Researchers and research managers must avoid any temptation to act in the role of clinician to the service user researcher, as this is inappropriate and undermining; professional and personal boundaries must be observed.

- Dissemination needs to take into account the service user audience as well as the research and other stakeholder audiences.

REFERENCES

Allam, S., Blyth, S., Fraser, A., Hodgson, S., Howes, J. and Newman, A. (2004) 'Our experience of collaborative research: Service users, carers and researchers work together to evaluate an assertive outreach service.' *Journal of Psychiatric and Mental Health Nursing 11*, 3, 365–373.

Beresford, P. (2003) 'User involvement in research: Exploring the challenges.' *Nursing Times Research 8*, 1, 36–45.

Consumers in NHS Research Support Unit (1999) *Involving Consumers in Research and Development in the NHS: Briefing Notes for Researchers.* London: Department of Health.

Department of Health (1998) *Health Research: What's in it for Consumers? Report of the Standing Advisory Committee on Consumer Involvement in the NHS Research and Development Programme.* London: Department of Health. Available at www. dh.gov.uk/en/Publicationsandstatistics/Publications/PublicationsPolicy andGuidance/DH_4002744, accessed on 12 May 2009.

Department of Health (1999) *Patient and Public Involvement in the New NHS.* London: Department of Health.

Department of Health (2000) *Working in Partnerships: Consumers in Research, Third Annual Report.* London: Department of Health.

Hanley, B. (2003) *Involving the Public in NHS, Public and Social Care Research: Briefing Notes for Researchers*, 2nd edn. Eastleigh: INVOLVE.

Joseph Rowntree Foundation (2005) *User Involvement in Research: Building on Experience and Developing Standards.* Findings, April, Ref. 0175. York: Joseph Rowntree Foundation. Available at www.jrf.org.uk/node/1332, accessed on 12 May 2009.

Lindow, V. (2001) 'Survivor Research.' In C. Newness, G. Holmes and C. Dunn (eds) *This is Madness Too. Critical Perspectives on Mental Health Services.* London: PCCS Books.

Lindow, V. (2002) 'How can survivor research make a difference, and what are the ethical issues? Being ethical, having influence.' *Open Mind 116*, July/August, 18–19.

Lockey, R., Sitzia, J., Gillingham, T., Millyard, J. *et al.* (2004) *Training for Service User Involvement in Health and Social Care Research: A Study of Training Provision and Participants' Experiences.* Eastleigh: INVOLVE.

Mental Health Research Network (2005) *Guidance for Good Practice: Service User Involvement in the UK.* London: Mental Health Research Network.

Ramon, S. (2000) 'Participative mental health research: Users and professional researchers working together.' *Mental Health Care 3,* 7, 224–228.

Rose, D. (2003) 'Collaborative research between users and professional: Peaks and pitfalls.' *Psychiatric Bulletin 27,* 11, 404–406.

Rose, D., Wykes, T. and Leese, M. (2004) 'Patients' perspectives on electroconvulsive therapy: a systematic review.' *British Medical Journal 326,* June, 1363–1366.

Royle, J., Steel, R., Hanley, B. and Bradburn, J. (2001) *Getting Involved in Research: A Guide for Consumers.* Eastleigh: Consumers in NHS Research Support Unit. Available from INVOLVE at http://invo.org.uk/pdfs/guide_for_consumers. pdf, accessed on 12 May 2009.

Stringer, E. (2004) *Action Research in Education.* Upper Slade River, NJ: Pearson Education.

Tilakaratna, S. (1990) *A Short Note on Participatory Research.* Caledonia Centre for Social Development. Available at www.caledonia.org.uk/research.htm, accessed on 12 May 2009.

Townsend, M. and Braithwaite, T. (2002) 'Mental health research: The value of user involvement.' *Journal of Mental Health 11,* 2, 117–119.

Trivedi, P. and Wykes, T. (2002) 'From passive subjects to equal partners.' *British Journal of Psychiatry 181,* 6, 468–472.

Wykes, T. (2003) 'Blue skies in the Journal of Mental Health? Consumers in research.' *Journal of Mental Health 12,* 1, 1–6.

CHAPTER 11

The Creative Involvement of Service Users in the Classroom

Philip Kemp

INTRODUCTION AND BACKGROUND

As the philosophy and imperative for user involvement has increasingly influenced mental health practice and service provision, there has been an inevitable pressure to address the implications of this for the education and training of mental health professionals and others who work in the mental health field. There have been significant calls for involving mental health service users in the education and training of mental health professionals over the years. The *National Service Framework for Mental Health* states that 'service users should be involved in planning, providing and evaluating education and training' (Department of Health 1999, p.109). The relationship between the mental health nurse and the user of mental health services was the central focus of a comprehensive review of mental health nursing (Department of Health 1994). The review made a specific recommendation that 'People who use services and their carers should participate in teaching and curriculum development' (Department of Health 1994, Recommendation 28). At the same time the report acknowledged that there is no consensus on how this should be achieved. This recommendation was replicated in a report about the training of mental health professionals (Sainsbury Centre for Mental Health 1997), although it too recognized that the 'difficult issue' of user involvement in education and training programmes has not been comprehensively addressed. The Chief Nursing Officer's review of mental health nursing recommended 'Higher education institutions to involve service users and carers in every aspect of education' including recruitment; curriculum planning; teaching and student assessment (Department of Health 2006, Recommendation 14). The Nursing and Midwifery Council now requires all nurse education programmes to involve service users in student recruitment, curriculum development, course delivery, student assessment and course monitoring.

The education and training of social workers has been influenced by similar expectations. Involving service users in social work education and its potential benefits is not new (Beresford 1994). The introduction of a new educational preparation for social workers, with a three-year degree course replacing a two-year diploma in 2002, provided an opportunity for a fundamental review of the nature of social work training. There is now a requirement for service users to be involved in the recruitment and training of social work students (Department of Health 2002). Each training institution has been provided with funds specifically for this purpose and there are developments within social work to formulate how service user involvement can be made effective, including the development of good practice guides (Levin 2004; Tew, Gell and Foster 2004). In addition to mental health nursing and social work, there is increasing activity in involving service users in the training of other mental health professional groups, including psychiatrists (see, for example, Hurren 2006; Ikkos 2003; Vijayakrishnan *et al.* 2006) and clinical psychologists (see, for example, Curle and Mitchell 2003; Goodbody *et al.* 2007).

However, despite a significant range of policy prescriptions, development of good practice guidelines, and some published examples of involvement initiatives, little is known about *how* and the extent to which user involvement in professional mental health education is being implemented (Repper and Breeze 2004, p.9). The challenge for providers of professional education and training is how to make user involvement a genuine reality and identify the potential benefits.

This chapter will describe a workshop approach to involving service users in the teaching and learning of student mental health nurses which proved to be a positive experience for both students and service users. The approach generated valuable insights into how best to achieve genuine service user participation in educational settings and demonstrated the 'added value' of involving service users. The methods described arose out of a larger participatory action research project (Kemp 2008) which aimed to explore and evaluate effective ways of involving service users in the educational activities within mental health nurse training and education (Kemp 2008). This chapter draws upon some of those experiences and findings.

INVOLVING SERVICE USERS IN PROFESSIONAL EDUCATION AND TRAINING

It has to be remembered that genuine, effective, safe and sustainable involvement of service users in classroom teaching and learning requires considerable levels of collaborative effort to reach a stage where it is possible to implement such an approach. Consideration needs to be given to the strategies employed to access service users interested in becoming involved. Thought also needs to be given about how to effectively engage service users in the process, planning and preparation to become involved, developing a session, debriefing and feedback arrangements after the session, practical considerations on the day of the session, and not least issues of payment. Systems, processes and training need to be established both to support service users and to support staff. All this suggests the need for a strategic approach to service user involvement in educational activities for it to be a success. Space limitations do not allow these important matters to be addressed in this chapter (for further help, see Beales *et al.* 2006; Campbell 2006; Repper and Breeze 2004). Here the focus will be specifically on the actual involvement of service users in the classroom.

CRITICAL ISSUES IN RELATION TO USE OF SERVICE USER 'TESTIMONIES' AS A TEACHING TOOL

A key aim of the author's research project on involving service users in teaching and learning (Kemp 2008) was to increase the numbers of service users involved and to widen the range of service users to include 'less confident' service users. One of the reasons for adopting a workshop approach is that what might be considered a 'conventional' understanding of user involvement in education was questioned. This focused on individual service users making a presentation, based on their own personal experiences, to a group of students usually followed by a question and answer session. A member of academic staff would normally be present to oversee the classroom management aspects of the session, such as introducing the service user and facilitating the question and answer session. Service users' presentations would generally be concerned with giving their 'stories'. Examples of such sessions typically included users' personal accounts of their experience of mental illness or some aspect of it such as hearing voices and their self-management, experiences of particular interventions, such as medication, or working in a user organization or advocacy role.

One of the benefits often cited for this form of contribution is that as professionals our understanding of psychological distress is partial and limited (Bracken and Thomas 2001; Double 2002). Diamond *et al.* (2003) argue that the inclusion of users' experiences and knowledge through service user involvement elaborates on this limited understanding of distress (Diamond *et al.* 2003, p.614). Personal testimonies, it is argued, also constitute a potential source of good practice 'where experience is not seen as subjective and irrelevant but a valuable evidence base' (May 2001, p.15). The importance of 'experiential knowledge' from service users to counterbalance the professional imperative of evidence-based practice is emphasized by Rose *et al.* (2004). Many of these writers have emphasized the importance of personal testimony in education and training as a contrast to the dominant discourse of psychiatry.

Students appear to value sessions where service users 'tell their story'. However, an evaluation suggested that the contribution to student learning by way of personal testimony can be problematic for a number of reasons. For example, it is evident that not all service users are comfortable with this approach and many are not confident enough to make individual presentations to a class of students. Some service users did not wish to give away too much of themselves, even if it had potential educational value. One service user, who had been involved in presenting his 'story' to students, nevertheless expressed ambivalent feelings about the role of personal testimony. He conceptualized the role of the service user in personal testimony as 'representing your vulnerability'. More pointedly he observed that 'My interest value is my illness – my freakishness'. It appeared that for some service users, there was a feeling that despite any positive contribution they might make to student learning, there was also a sense that this interest value was their separateness because of their experience of mental illness. This has the potential risk of increasing stigmatization and reinforcing stereotypical conceptions of mental illness.

Even when service users did feel comfortable about sharing their experiences, there could be unintended consequences for the service user that needed to be responded to as a result. For example, one service user had been invited to talk to a group of students about her experiences of self-harm. This service user enjoyed undertaking the session and students gave warm and positive feedback. However, the experience nevertheless left her feeling 'exhausted' and 'deflated'. She had no regrets about the session and indeed some months later repeated the talk with another group of students.

Another potential problem is that in telling their story, service users might be drawn along by the occasion and inadvertently reveal more about themselves than they intended. A further point made by several service users is that they did not like repeating the same session too often as for them it paralleled their experience of mental health services in the sense that in their contacts with mental health professionals, they frequently have to repeat their story in the process of professional 'history taking'.

Other service users reported that they found some 'therapeutic' value in telling their story. The therapeutic value appeared to be not so much because of cathartic processes but because there was a sense of fulfilment at 'contributing to something worthwhile' in the form of student nurse education and training.

Despite the apparent benefits of individual user presentations, lack of confidence in making individual presentations to students; discomfort with the idea of personal testimony; the emotional labour of sharing your story with an audience of students (essentially strangers) resulted, therefore, in looking increasingly to the use of workshop-style sessions alongside individual presentations and other approaches to teaching and learning.

THE USE OF WORKSHOP APPROACHES

Classes of students were divided into subgroups of four or five. One or more service users would join each subgroup and participate with students in a set activity. The format for the workshop sessions typically involved setting students tasks such as developing responses to practice-based scenarios. The intention was that a more informed response would emerge with a service user perspective contributing to the discussion. Each subgroup would feed back to the larger group and further discussion was generated.

An example of the scenarios used for these sessions was a session entitled Practice Dilemmas that was used with third year students. The idea was to get them to think through the decision-making process when confronted in practice with challenging, yet common, situations. Such encounters can be seen as characteristic of many aspects of mental health practice. Practitioners are confronted with situations where decisions are not straightforward, or where there is no clear evidence base to draw on. Instead practice decisions have to be based on a judgement. Such judgements are open to question and the issue is how to make the 'best' judgement in a given situation. Many things might help inform the decision-making process and a central consideration should be service user perspectives.

An example of the sort of practice dilemma used in the workshop-based sessions involving service users is given below. Mental health nursing students, when given such a scenario, will often focus only on the illness and treatment of the 'patient'. Service users will draw their attention to the 'person' who – in this scenario – is a mother and will have concerns about her children.

> Mrs Davis, aged 38, was admitted informally to an inpatient unit on Thursday afternoon. She had been experiencing depression and was admitted after taking a large overdose of her antidepressant medication. She had taken the overdose in the morning after taking her two children, aged 8 and 10 years, to school. Her husband, with the help of his mother, was looking after her children. It is now 7pm on Friday and Mrs Davis has packed her bags saying that she wants to go home.

This approach works particularly well if there is a small group of service users who regularly work together within workshop sessions and can form a user 'teaching team', building up confidence in themselves and accumulating experience in the delivery of the session.

One of the aspects that service users found more comfortable about participating in workshop sessions was that it did not necessarily entail sharing their personal histories in any great detail. Service users were able to self-regulate how much of their 'story' they wished to share. What they were able to do was to impart a service user perspective into the discussions and help students think more deeply about how user sensitive their actions might be and incorporate this into their professional decision-making.

In addition some service users felt more comfortable about being involved in small group discussions with four or five students rather than addressing a whole class. They were not expected to feed back to the larger group during the feedback part of the session (although they often did). Interestingly the feedback component generated further discussion and most service users involved made additional comments to the larger group as part of this process, as in time they generally felt comfortable and safe to do so. There was also an element of mutual support among service users in contributing in this shared approach.

CHARACTERISTICS AND POTENTIAL BENEFITS OF WORKSHOP-BASED SESSIONS

In the ongoing observation and evaluation of this approach to involving service users in the classroom, a high level of agreement was identified between students, staff and service users about a number of factors that were considered as contributing to the 'added value' of involving service users in the teaching and learning of mental health nurses. Seven key elements are summarized here and discussed below:

1. Workshop-based sessions create the conditions for more open dialogue between students and service users.

2. Service user perspectives are incorporated in students' consideration of practice-based scenario responses.

3. Students reappraise their perceptions of service users.

4. Power dynamics between students and service users are changed.

5. Students gain insights and understanding that are not accessible in the practice setting.

6. Developmental discussions are characterized by a step-wise process of 'structured conversations'.

7. Sessions involving service users are consistently positively evaluated.

Workshop-based sessions create the conditions for more open dialogue between students and service users

Students and service users interacted together within the classroom in distinctive ways: in their general style of communication students adopted a respectful approach; they were polite and appreciative; and they appeared to interact positively as a result of the relatively informal setting compared to their interactions with service users in practice settings. Where opportunities arose, they were able to engage in 'non-professionalized' conversations and talk about 'ordinary', everyday matters.

This approach consistently promoted high levels of engagement in the workshop activity itself. Many teachers in higher education will have experienced students displaying different levels of engagement in set tasks and a challenge for teachers is to ensure that they facilitate genuine learning opportunities when using a workshop approach. Where service users are involved students engage more fully in the activity.

Thus the workshop sessions acted as a vehicle for promoting interaction and dialogue between students and service users. Students frequently reported that they do not have the time or the opportunity to interact in the same way with service users when they are undertaking practice placements. This is certainly consistent with research and evaluations into the levels of nurse and service user interaction in inpatient settings (see, for example, Ricketts 1996; Whittington and McLaughlin 2000).

The dialogue between students and service users within the classroom created a 'communicative space' which previously did not exist, or at least only to a very limited extent. Students and service users were brought together in a specific social context different from their usual interface, with different expectations and for different purposes. This social context, within the classroom, influenced the nature of the dialogue and the way service users and students engaged with each other. Students consistently reported that they felt able to discuss issues which were not possible within the practice setting. Such sessions facilitated not only the expression of 'service user voices' but also an *alternative* voice for students in their interactions with service users. Students also felt freed up to speak in a more open way compared to their interactions with service users in the practice setting.

This evaluation suggests that in practice environments students experience some inhibitions in their interactions with service users because of organizational pressures and professional roles. However, in the classroom such inhibitions appear to be loosened, resulting in more open dialogue. This is one of the factors consistently cited by students as a positive benefit of involving service users in their education and training.

Service user perspectives are incorporated in students' consideration of practice-based scenario responses

The workshop sessions helped students look at practice situations from different angles that incorporated service users' perspectives. They served as a method of helping students to appreciate service user perspectives in a way that is difficult to do by other means. The approach recognizes service users as experts in their own experience, a source of expertise that teachers do not necessarily possess. There is an authenticity about involving service users which can convey user perspectives more powerfully than a lecturer or textbook.

Students were facilitated to reflect on the service users' unique circumstances. Students were prompted to consider issues that they might otherwise not have thought of. Perspectives of service users add another layer of learning in the classroom beyond lectures and reading.

Students reappraise their perceptions of service users

In the evaluations many students commented on how their experience of interacting with service users in the workshop sessions conflicted with their preconceptions of service users. The high levels of engagement between students and service users and the relative informality of workshop-based sessions helped undermine stereotyped perceptions of service users and enabled students to appreciate that service users were, as one student remarked, 'no different from us', that service users often had careers, families and could speak articulately and insightfully about mental health practices as well as about their own personal experiences.

For many students their previous experience of service users was solely within the practice environment, often when service users were experiencing a period of crisis or heightened distress, which arguably skews students' perceptions of people who have experienced mental health difficulties. The attraction of the workshop approach described here is that it provides opportunities for face-to-face interaction with service users without many of the distortions that the structure of professional practice tends to impose. This process was further helped by sharing break times and the opportunities for informal conversations that this afforded. Being able to see service users as people rather than 'patients' is an important potential benefit. The opportunity to engage with service users outside of the professionally structured practice environment was seen to be of high potential value.

Power dynamics between students and service users are changed

The power dynamics between students and service users in the classroom were more equally balanced, if not reversed, compared with the relationships experienced in practice settings. Students' comments in this respect also seem to relate this to the professional role they are expected to adopt in practice that emphasizes their separation as 'staff' from 'patients'. Observations of student–user interaction discussed above reinforced perceptions of the realignment of power relations in so far as students tended to relate to service users as 'teachers' or 'experts' in a situation where students and service users were working together in shared activities. This offered a means of providing a structure to student and service user interactions and is a theme discussed in more detail below. Undertaking shared tasks in this way, where there was a mutual searching for an appropriate outcome, also contributed to the realignment of power relations in the classroom compared to practice.

Students gain insights and understanding that are not accessible in the practice setting

The workshop-based sessions involving service users demonstrated the potential benefits of students learning with service users *outside* of the practice environment. While approximately 50 per cent of the students' educational programme is undertaken in practice placements, the nature and conditions of the dialogue in the workshop sessions meant that students were able to elicit knowledge, understanding and insights that they would not have been able to elicit in the practice environment. The nature of the more open dialogue and the opportunities for this in workshop sessions described above underline the significance of the differences in the way students interact with service users in the classroom compared to the practice environment. As one student commented, service users are able to draw upon 'practical experiences which professionals might not be sensitive enough to discover'.

While students perceived service users interacting more freely in the classroom compared to practice settings, students said that they themselves were also able to interact more freely. The openness of the interactions in the workshop sessions was a mutual experience between students and service users. The evidence of high levels of engagement between students and service users discussed above lends support to student perceptions of openness in themselves.

Students frequently attributed the more open dialogue to being away from the constraints imposed by organizational factors within the practice setting (for example, ward environments) and professional roles when interacting with service users in the practice setting. There appeared to be recognition that the students' professional role acted as an inhibiting factor in their interactions with service users in practice settings. Interacting in a setting outside of the practice environment appeared to be important in promoting open dialogue. To some extent both students and service users were interacting 'out of role' within the classroom. The relaxation in relationships with service users compared to practice, which students described, was further reinforced by observing students and service users interacting during breaks in the session.

Perhaps more controversially it has to be acknowledged that not all staff within the practice settings represent ideal role models for student mental health practitioners. In this respect the involvement of service users in the classroom might be considered as a counterpoint to some mentors encountered by students in practice. Involving service users in the classroom is a way of helping students reflect on their relationships with service users in practice.

Developmental discussions are characterized by a step-wise process of 'structured conversations'

The adoption of user perspectives in problem solving the workshop practice dilemmas appeared to develop in an incremental fashion as the discussions involving service users evolved during the session. The *process* of discussion appeared to be of equal significance, if not more, than the outcome of workshop discussions in respect of the conclusions reached in relation to the workshop scenarios. As one service user observed:

> To begin with students came up with stock answers. They were bogged down in procedures: contact the duty doctor; section the patient. It came as a revelation that you might want to talk to the patient first.

Typically students were initially concerned with 'gathering information' rather than analysing or reflecting on the scenarios and relied on 'stock answers' or 'applying a drill' in the discussions. It was observed that students had a tendency to adopt procedural responses. However, as the discussion developed, they gained the ability to uncover the complexities and subtleties of practice situations including how issues of stigma might be inadvertently reinforced.

Service users also found that they took on a facilitating role within subgroups in order to steer students towards thinking about user perspectives within the scenarios, for example, helping them think harder about how service users might feel in the situation under discussion. In this sense the workshop discussions acted as 'structured conversations' which appeared to capture the informality of interaction but at the same time the guiding role of service user input.

Overall, the process of reaching the answers included the following ways in which user perspectives were infused into the discussion:

- Assumptions could be corrected.

- Issues or ideas that had not occurred to students could be pointed out.

- The subtleties of situations could be identified.

- A different way of looking at a situation could be explained.

Through the process of discussion and the step-wise development of responses to workshop scenarios, students appeared to move from 'procedural interventions' to a gradual accommodation of user perspectives.

Sessions involving service users are consistently positively evaluated

Evidence of the benefits of user involvement is demonstrated by students' positive feedback, which expressed high levels of engagement and enjoyment. Most teachers would feel some satisfaction about the success of the teaching and learning they are responsible for with such consistently positive evaluations by students.

CONCLUSION

A number of potential benefits have been identified for involving service users in workshop-based teaching and learning sessions in the classroom. While a range of approaches can usefully be adopted, workshop-style sessions as a general approach are an effective means for involving a wider range of service users, many of whom feel more comfortable with small-group discussions that do not necessarily require a detailed sharing of their personal history of mental health difficulties.

There are also indications that not only do students value these sessions but also there is some added value for student learning. The experience of involving service users in workshop-based teaching and learning sessions in the classroom suggests that students interact with service users in the classroom in distinctive ways. The classroom constitutes a 'communicative space', relatively free of the professional and organizational pressures found in the practice environment which might impact on student and service user interactions.

Thus alongside 'theory' and 'practice', it is suggested here that there can be significant benefits to professional education and training from a 'third sphere' of learning. A third sphere of learning is essentially the provision of learning opportunities for students in the form of direct face-to-face engagement with service users *outside* of the practice setting which provides an opportunity for learning that is neither readily available in practice nor accessible in conventional theory-based classroom learning. Service user input in the context of the workshop sessions potentially provides a valuable form of learning. It is more than simply including 'invited experts' or simply to add additional colour to a topic. It is not 'icing on the cake' nor an added extra to enrich the course. From this perspective, user involvement in the ways described in this chapter is viewed as a fundamental necessity for student learning and understanding of user experiences and the application of user perspectives to how they approach practice.

At the same time, although such sessions with service users are inherently about practice they are not 'in practice'. They are consequently disengaged from professional practice or organizational influences that structure interactions and relationships in practice. Students are interacting with service users directly but not in a professional practice context. The 'rules of engagement' between students and service users in the classroom that is within the 'third sphere' of learning are qualitatively different from those found in the practice environment. The more challenging issue is that benefits could lead to lasting changes in practice.

GOOD PRACTICE GUIDANCE FOR INVOLVING SERVICE USERS

- A range of different approaches for involving service users in educational activities should be available to promote opportunities for wide participation.

- Involving small groups of service users in workshop approaches is particularly effective in promoting high levels of informal interaction between students and service users which has the potential to change students' views of users.

- Appropriate support arrangements, including preparation before an activity and debriefing after an educational event, need to be in place to ensure that the experience is a satisfying one for service user, students and academic staff.

- Service users want and can benefit from feedback about their participation and this needs to be built into the process of involvement.

REFERENCES

Beales, A., Beresford, P., Hitchon, G., Westra, A. and Basset, T. (2006) *Service Users Together: A Guide for Involvement* . London: Together.

Beresford, P. (1994) *Changing the Culture: Involving Service Users in Social Work Education.* London: Central Council of Education and Training in Social Work.

Bracken, P. and Thomas, P. (2001) 'Postpsychiatry: A new direction in mental health.' *British Medical Journal 322*, 724–727.

Campbell, P. (2006) *Some Things You Should Know about User/Survivor Action – A MIND Resource Pack.* London: MIND.

Curle, C. and Mitchell, A. (2003) 'Hand in hand: User and carer involvement in training clinical psychologists.' *Clinical Psychology 33*, 12–15.

Department of Health (1994) *Working in Partnership – A Collaborative Approach to Care: Report of the Mental Health Nursing Review Team.* London: HMSO.

Department of Health (1999) *National Service Framework for Mental Health.* London: Department of Health.

Department of Health (2002) *Requirements for the Degree in Social Work.* London: Department of Health.

Department of health (2006) *From Values to Action: The Chief Nursing Officer's Review of Mental Health Nursing.* London: Department of Health.

Diamond, B., Parkin, G., Morris, K., Bettinis, J. and Bettesworth, C. (2003) 'User involvement: Substance or spin?' *Journal of Mental Health 12*, 6, 613–626.

Double, D. (2002) 'The limits of psychiatry.' *British Medical Journal 324*, 900–904.

Goodbody, L., Haywood, M., Hulttum, S. and Riddell, B. (2007) *Integrating Service User and Carer Involvement into Clinical Psychology Training.* Higher Educational Academy Psychology Network Final Report, Canterbury: Centre for Applied Social and Psychological Development, Canterbury Christchurch University.

Hurren, K. (2006) 'Impact on trainees of involving users and carers in teaching.' *Meriden Programme 2*, 9, 11–13.

Kemp, P. (2008) *User Involvement in the Education and Training of Student Mental Health Nurses in the Classroom.* Unpublished PhD thesis. London: South Bank University.

Ikkos, G. (2003) 'Engaging patients as teachers of clinical interview skills.' *Psychiatric Bulletin 27*, 8, 312–315.

Levin, E. (2004) *Involving Service Users and Carers in Social Work Education.* Resource Guide No. 2. London: Social Care Institute for Excellence.

May, R. (2001) 'Crossing the "them and us" barriers: An inside perspective on user involvement in clinical psychology.' *Clinical Psychology Forum 150*, 14–17.

Repper, J. and Breeze, J. (2004) *A Review of the Literature on User and Carer Involvement in the Education and Training of Health Care Professionals.* Sheffield: Sheffield Health and Social Care Research Consortium.

Ricketts, T. (1996) 'General satisfaction and satisfaction with nursing communication on an adult psychiatric ward.' *Journal of Advanced Nursing 24,* 3, 479–487.

Rose, D., Fleischmann, P., Tonkiss, F., Campbell, P. and Wykes, T. (2004) *User and Carer Involvement in Change Management in a Mental Health Context: Review of the Literature.* Report to the National Co-ordinating Centre for NHS Service Delivery and Organisation Research and Development (NCCSDO). London: NCCSDO.

Sainsbury Centre for Mental Health (1997) *Pulling Together: The Future Roles and Training of Mental Health Staff.* London: Sainsbury Centre for Mental Health.

Tew, J., Gell, C. and Foster, S. (2004) *Learning from Experience: Involving Service Users and Carers in Mental Health Education and Training.* Nottingham: Higher Education Academy, National Institute for Mental Health in England and Trent Workforce Development Confederation.

Vijayakrishnan, A., Rutherford, J., Miller, S. and Drummond, L.M. (2006) 'Service user involvement in training: The trainee's view.' *Psychiatric Bulletin 30,* 8, 303–305.

Whittington, D. and McLaughlin, C. (2000) 'Finding time for patients: An exploration of nurses' time allocation in an acute psychiatric setting.' *Journal of Psychiatric and Mental Health Nursing 7,* 3, 259–268.

CHAPTER 12

Meeting the Challenge of Working with Young Care Leavers in Delivering Social Work Training

Tom Wilks and Liz Green

INTRODUCTION

The title of this chapter poses as many questions as it sets out to answer. It could be assumed that young people are challenging to work with and this chapter could then analyse how to meet these challenges from the perspective of adult professionals. Alternatively, the focus could be to consider the challenges that confront young care leavers' involvement in aspects of their lives. We will attempt to span both of these questions in the context of involving young care leavers in social work education in the UK, drawing on a specific example of how this has been successfully implemented.

We begin our discussion with an exploration of the reasons for user involvement at both the broader policy level and at the institutional level. We then move on to examine why we saw the involvement of young people with experience of the care system as being a specific priority. There were many practical and educational challenges presented in engaging and involving young people in the training of social workers; we look at these and then finally reflect upon the outcomes of that involvement focusing upon what we have learnt and how it has shaped our perspectives on mental health, pedagogy and the place of service users in social work education.

Within the broader context of user involvement and participation in mental health services it is crucial that the perspectives of people with mental health problems from across the age span are represented. Our intention throughout this chapter is to emphasize that those experiencing mental distress are not a homogeneous group despite being faced with many similar difficulties. Young people leaving care face a number of problems which are particular to their circumstances. Our motivation in working with them was in part to broaden our students' overall understanding of this extremely vulnerable group who 'are at high risk of developing mental health disorders which often persist into adult life' with 'little if any provision of mental health services which target their needs' (Mental Health Foundation 2001, p.82).

CONTEXT OF SERVICE USER INVOLVEMENT

One key factor influencing our decision to involve young people was the increased emphasis placed upon service user involvement (Department of Health 2000) and the changes in social work education in the UK, ushered in by the General Social Care Council (GSCC) (Department of Health 2002). The advent of the GSCC itself marked a change in how professional social work practice in the UK was conceived, codifying both the skills and value bases of the profession, and more closely aligning it with related professional groups such as nursing (Banks 2004).

One of the ways in which a distinctive social work orientation to the process of professionalization was maintained was through this consistent concern with service user involvement. Service user involvement was seen as important in the planning and development of services. Over and above this, however, the aspiration of the GSCC was that involvement would also help remodel the relationship between social worker and service user into one where service users had greater power and were more able to influence the nature and process of social work intervention. These principles of service user involvement were manifested in the requirements that universities had to meet with the advent of a new degree in social work in 2002 (see Chapter 11). For us, thinking about how to involve young people, a key end goal was to encourage social work students to adopt more empowering approaches to practice. Furthermore, we were keen that young people should be able to influence both the content of teaching and the style in which it would be delivered.

We were aware of a number of risks attendant upon the involvement of service users, many of which have been well documented elsewhere

(Beresford 2001; Croft and Beresford 1993). There is a clear concern that involvement of service users may be tokenistic with their input parachuted into existing programmes of study, without any change to either the overall content or delivery of the programme concerned. Here service users may be presented as consumers of the services they receive, with little power to shape services, or to become equal participants in relationships with professional care providers.

We were also keen to avoid the personal testimony model (Levin 2004; Manthorpe 2000; see also Chapter 11) of learning and teaching where service users are brought into academic institutions to tell their stories. Although we were well aware of the power of these stories, we were concerned that they emphasize the difference in experience between service users, students and academics, and locate service user experience outside the mainstream of teaching and learning.

Basset, Campbell and Anderson (2006) detail ten barriers found in their mental health training research that prevent the involvement of service users and carers in learning and teaching. These barriers, also found in other literature (Levin 2004), can be applied to all service user groups. They include the following: the reluctance of professionals to give up power; seeing users as 'problems' rather than as valued contributors; a tokenistic approach; the use of jargon; excuses for the non-inclusion of service users and carers; reluctance to acknowledge that their contribution is as important and not inferior to 'academic' knowledge, and the lack of payment and support for service user and carer contributors. So key goals for us embarking upon the process of involving young people in teaching and learning were to overcome these barriers and to try to adopt approaches which shared power (in so far as this is possible) and allowed young people to challenge us and our students.

INVOLVING YOUNG CARE LEAVERS IN SOCIAL WORK EDUCATION

We have identified two connected reasons for involving young people from the public care system in social work education. The first relates to the disempowerment of young people who have been in care, the second to the importance of young people's perspectives on mental health being addressed in social work training.

Young people who have been in care are a particularly disempowered group (Hill *et al.* 2004), who are often excluded from the processes of decision-making about services in general and more specifically about their own care. Levin (2004) provides a comprehensive guide to the involvement of service users and carers in social work education. She brings together a wide range of literature which explores the development of service user and carer involvement in social work education as well as guidelines and examples of good practice. However, what is clearly missing from the overview is the voice of young care leavers. This poses the question of whether this group are too challenging for such involvement, inaccessible due to confidentiality or lacking a loud enough voice demanding that they be heard. Within the Children Act 1989 (HM Government 1989) and the *United Nations Convention on the Rights of the Child* (United Nations 1989) there is a requirement to respect children's views. Government guidelines (Department of Health 2002, 2004) advocate making 'particular efforts' to ensure that looked after children, as a 'frequently excluded group', are supported and encouraged to give their views and to be involved in decision-making. Davies and Wright (2008) identify in their review of literature concerning looked after children's views of mental health services, that clinicians may be reluctant to engage in discussions with looked after children due to their vulnerability concerning insecure attachments. Davies and Wright (2008) review a range of studies which have shown that, with support, looked after children can provide feedback on services (Dance and Rushton 2005; Potter, Holmes and Barton 2002; Prior, Lynch and Glaser 1999). The suggestion is therefore that looked after children are frequently not given the opportunity to become involved in providing feedback and thus are prevented from having their voices heard. This applies equally to their exclusion from social work education.

A key challenge in working with young care leavers is therefore ensuring that their voice is heard. Rightly so, the details of children and young people in care are not available to the public. This means that for the sake of research, consultation or involvement in social work education, a complex process of consent is required which surprisingly, is 'less defined than in health settings' (Davies and Wright 2008) and prevents the views of looked after children being represented in research and social work training. They suggest one decision-making body in loco parentis to overcome this problem.

Voice of the Child in Care and other organizations have provided avenues for their voices to be heard in the media, within organizations and via the internet. However, the more traditional voices of adults with mental and physical disabilities tend to dominate and lead. Children and young people's position in the background may be due to their place in society and the reluctance of adults to take them seriously.

Because of this we were keen to establish approaches to learning and teaching that helped make young people more powerful and gave them expertise. We also hoped that they would benefit from the process. It is increasingly recognized (Sanders and Munford 2007) that relationships between service users and educators ought to be reciprocal whereby both service user and academic institution benefit.

We were also acutely aware that the issue of mental health is one that is often addressed from the adult perspective. For example, anthologies concerned with service user experience are often almost exclusively focused on adults (see, for example, Read and Reynolds 1997); yet we also know from research how damaging the impact of the care system can be on both children's and adult's mental health (Russell, Viner and Taylor 2005).

The involvement of young people in learning and teaching in social work gives a more holistic view of mental health and allows students to view this aspect of human experience from a life-course focused, developmental perspective. So often teaching in mental health emphasizes difference and deficit models. Models of mental well-being for those in the care system emphasize resilience (Gilligan 2000) and their involvement in learning and teaching embodies this concept. The development of young people can thus be seen within a lifespan perspective and not as abnormal and medical. Stein (2005) suggests that those in care should be seen, in common with all young people, as embarking on a shared process of development, which although it has a different starting point within the care system, has a common end in adulthood. The mental health needs of young people, particularly those who have experienced the care system, can be complex. While they include difficulties with mood and disordered thinking, key focuses of adult mental health services, they also span a wide range of other issues ranging from substance misuse and self-harm to problems with eating and diet (Richardson and Joughin 2001). Being confronted with this complexity helps students move away from a simple binary conception of a mental health or illness divide towards a more complex understanding of mental well-being within a social and developmental context.

Young care leavers not only have been through identity development during adolescence (Erikson 1971; Marcia 1966) and undergone the crises which can occur during that time, but also they have often lacked the support to allow them to achieve a positive self-image and sustain relationships. Gilligan (2000) emphasizes the need for positive relationships at any age in the lifespan, and for young care leavers in particular, because this can help improve self-image. In addressing this group of young people's mental health needs, social work students need to be aware of both developmental issues related to attachment and the impact of often traumatic life experience. The practice implications therefore are for social workers to pay attention to the need for young people to have people in their lives, who take an interest in them, who will listen to, care for and love them. This will bolster their self-esteem. One of our hopes was that involving young service users with experience of the care system in social work education would focus students' attention on these needs so crucial to the well-being of young people.

THE PRACTICAL AND EDUCATIONAL CHALLENGES OF INVOLVING YOUNG CARE LEAVERS

Goldsmiths College, University of London, had a history of adult service user participation in teaching and learning but the voice of children and young people came solely through videos and written commentaries produced by other organizations. Approaching young care leavers in order to consult on the new degree was a substantial departure and challenge. Initial contact appeared to be straightforward when a local voluntary sector organization agreed to a meeting with a group of young people. However, it became clear that we would need to be liaising with the local authority Leaving Care Team, who refer young people to this agency. Following a further meeting with the head of service for the borough, it was agreed that all young care leavers would be given the opportunity to take part in the consultation.

Approximately 200 packs of information were prepared by the university and distributed resulting in a group of five interested young people. Since two were under 18 years of age, consent for their involvement was established and an initial meeting with the young people undertaken at the social services Leaving Care department. This whole process was time consuming, and at times frustrating, but reflects the problems identified by Davies and Wright (2008).

Once the formalities had finally been completed, the consultation about the social work curriculum took the form of a focus group over five sessions, the subject of each being the areas identified by the GSCC (selection, teaching and learning, curriculum, assessment and management) and the young people were asked to consider materials to be used within all aspects of the proposed programmes. We used the focus group method as a model for the sessions as it offered a flexible and user-led approach which we hoped would make the service users' experience of this consultation process an empowering one (Linhorst 2002). With permission from the participants, the sessions were recorded to avoid note-taking dominating and disrupting the involvement of university staff.

Consideration was given to the differing circumstances of the young care leavers including income, child care responsibilities and housing, when making arrangements for meetings and making contact. All the young people received expenses for their time and travel and were provided with a meal of their choice during the session. Again there were challenges to arranging the meetings, including timekeeping and difficulties in keeping in contact, so a substantial level of support was needed from staff. It was essential to be flexible and to understand the situations in which these young people found themselves, such as bed and breakfast accommodation, debt and sometimes difficult relationships with peers.

OUTCOMES OF INVOLVEMENT

The resulting feedback from the young care leavers for course development was dynamic and exciting and acted as a springboard for new developments in service user and carer involvement. Three of the young people remained involved with the programmes following the consultation, having found the process interesting, engaging and empowering. They had many criticisms (and some praise) for their many social workers and wanted their voices heard in social work education. One key idea which shaped the service users' input into the project, and which became something of a mantra for the young people in critiquing our approaches to teaching and learning, was what we might call 'the person is not a case' approach. As recipients of social work input, many of the young people had experienced frequent changes of social worker and of being treated as 'cases' approached in a bureaucratic way by professionals, with little regard for individuality or need. 'The person is not the case' idea was identified by the young people involved in the project as a central feature of the training materials used to look at working with young care leavers, both video materials and case studies. Young people were highly critical of traditional video materials using actors that often present a narrow view of young people's lives focusing primarily on their interactions with professionals from a *professional* perspective, ignoring their wider worlds. Young people are often presented as non-challenging and receptive to social work input.

The next stage was to enable these young people to continue their curriculum development work so funding was identified by the university to produce original videos or DVDs whereby the young people could create materials which better reflected their experience of care. The young care leavers wanted genuine voices to be heard and to challenge the audience whether they were students, educators, social workers or policy makers. The videos they produced were conceived and scripted by the three young people and were filmed by a staff member. The young people presented their experience of care and fictional scenarios based around the review process. In these scenarios young people were shown behaving in an assertive way, challenging some of the approaches and attitudes adopted by professionals, providing a clear contrast with videos previously used on the course. The material provided a more complex and rounded account of young people in care, which, while acknowledging the challenge of being in care, also emphasized areas of young people's lives of value to them but often disregarded by social workers (the importance of friendships with peers for example), and focused on young people's resilience.

Student feedback on the videos showed that, although they may have felt uncomfortable or shocked, they appreciated hearing a real service user's voice; it challenged their assumptions about children in care and demonstrated the power of professionals. The following student comment is a good illustration of this:

> I think the young service user involvement is a very important and innovative step – I found it to be a humbling experience – where we might get carried away in our ideas and theories, this kept our feet on the ground.

Students particularly valued the way in which videos produced by young care leavers were an active demonstration of their expertise (expertise through experience) in relation to the public care system as a whole. Again students' comments show how important this aspect of the video was for them: 'I was surprised by the young person's confidence and self-esteem, which negates my opinions of looked after children' (Barnett *et al.* 2005).

When it came to putting what they had learnt from the video material into practice, students highlighted a number of key points, both general and more specifically related to the review process. The material enabled students to understand the importance of workers being clear about their responsibilities when working in multidisciplinary partnerships. It also served to emphasize the value of adopting a consistent approach when working with young people. In respect of reviewing the needs of those in care, the video helped make students more attentive to the importance of an effective process of preparation in which young people themselves actively participate, when their care is reviewed. Students' awareness was heightened about how young service users can easily be excluded from discussions within reviews and how intimidating a meeting of professionals can be for them. The video demonstrates the critical role played by the chairperson in review meetings and how when this role is effectively executed it can help young people's voices come to the fore. Another critical aspect of the students' learning from these materials was that all these issues have a broader resonance for all service users with mental health needs.

Subsequently the videos were used on the social work courses as part of a study unit concerning planning for children in care. Goldsmiths' social work courses employ problem-based learning as the main teaching and learning strategy and service user and carer involvement provided an important additional contribution to the optimal outcome of producing qualified social workers who understand the complexities of good practice (Green and Wilks 2009).

Two of the young people were particularly keen to remain involved, not only to make a further video or DVD with adult service users and carers, but also to take part in dissemination via conferences (Barnett *et al.* 2005; Kelsey *et al.* 2004) and consultations including service users and carers (Braye and Preston-Shoot 2006). The main challenges presented to the young people and social work staff concerned finance and child care. These were generally surmountable but required time and patience since those organizing conferences would initially not commit to financing child care, which excluded young care leavers with children. The young people also needed support when planning their presentations including the use of presentation aids for the event. For one of the young women, this has led to an increase in confidence which has allowed her to teach sessions at the university and apply for adult education courses to further her career. Her daughter has also been able to see her mother taking a leading role in conferences, thus providing a role model for her future development.

REFLECTIONS ON THE OUTCOMES OF THE YOUNG CARE LEAVERS' INVOLVEMENT

In order to move forward in practice, we have reflected upon what has been learned from our work with young care leavers and how it has impacted upon us as educators. We have increasingly recognized the important insights that young people bring which have broadened our (and students') understanding of mental health. To involve young people in learning and teaching successfully we have had to be attentive to issues of pedagogy, expand our understanding of our roles as teachers and focus on the reciprocal benefits for service users which come through involvement.

The strength and resilience of the young people we found remarkable. They were open and vocal about their experiences in care and both showed how vulnerable they have been and can be and how their resilience has helped them survive the child care system. They shared their experiences of loneliness, despair and low self-esteem with students and social work staff. They talked of how they had overcome some of these problems using state services, friends and family and their own ingenuity. Broad (2005) explored the experiences of care leavers whose education had been disrupted; they had been bullied, provided with poor accommodation and had little money. He identified these experiences as affecting their well-being and health and found that many used drink and drugs to make themselves feel better. The young people in Broad's (2005) study also considered that their mental health depended upon the respect and care provided by others.

For students this focus on resilience was important and gave them the opportunity to begin to conceptualize mental health beyond the confines of a narrow medical model. The young care leavers at Goldsmiths were clear that the problems which had necessitated their entry into care had frequently not been addressed and had often been exacerbated by failures of the system. Those factors which should contribute to resilience such as the provision of stability, a good quality education and a sense of identity, thus leading on to a supported transition to independence, had generally been missing. Without adequate support systems in place, young care leavers will be vulnerable and may put themselves in high risk situations. According to Stein (2005, p.33)' 'care should be at one end of a common developmental journey from being in care to becoming an adult'. We were aware of being part of this process and that it was necessary to try to demonstrate how social work can contribute to a positive outcome. Being reliable, respectful and empowering were therefore central to our relationships with the young care leavers with whom we were working. We also had to try to understand the pressures being experienced by these young people in their lives if we wanted to integrate their expert knowledge and experience into social work programmes and improve future practice.

It is something of a truism that in planning teaching and learning educators need to be aware of both the content and style or mode of delivery. The experience of working with this group of young service users brought home to us the intricate and symbiotic link between the two. The way in which we were able to use young care leavers' materials within the framework of problem-based learning (Burgess 1992; Burgess and Jackson 1990) played a crucial part in their effectiveness as tools for learning and teaching. The use of case studies offered young service users subject matter which they could critique, and develop. Additionally it enabled young service users to contribute to any given cycle of problem-based learning by acting as expert advisers to students on the plans for care they developed in relation to the case examples. As in the example described in Chapter 11, the employment of users as consultants in case-based learning moved involvement away from a personal testimony towards an approach premised on the idea of service users as experts through experience (Green and Wilks 2009).

For those teaching in social work education, the involvement of young service users demands a new set of skills and new approaches to learning and teaching as part of a team. For us it involved a complex process of contacting and liaising with local organizations offering support to looked after children. That liaison (and the ongoing provision of feedback about the project) continued on after the group of young service users was established. This activity had more in common with community development than learning and teaching. Forming a team with the young people to complete the projects on which we were working together meant adopting roles which extended beyond conventional relationships and roles in learning and teaching.

We have reflected upon the impact this small-scale project may have had on the lives of the young people. For the young care leavers, the involvement in such an activity can boost their resilience (Lockey *et al.* 2004). It can contribute to increased confidence and self-esteem as well as a realization that others value the voices of service users and carers. We enabled them to be part of conference presentations and research activity and witnessed how, with encouragement, they could present their views to a wider audience, where their challenging material could be shared. Our work became a reciprocal relationship where all concerned benefited and learned. This is in line with the Quality Assurance Agency (QAA) subject benchmark statement for social work (QAA 2000, 2008) which states that when 'providing services, social workers should engage with service users and carers in ways that are characterized by openness, reciprocity, mutual accountability and explicit recognition of the powers of the social worker and the legal context of intervention' (QAA 2000, p.11) and elaborated upon within academic literature (Dominelli 2004). We have seen how this reciprocal relationship between student, staff and service user has challenged views concerning the involvement of young people in consultations and research exercises. It has allowed their voice to be heard in other forums such as accreditation exercises, thus shifting power and moving the social work education agenda to include that of the service user (Arnstein 1969; Hart 1992).

CONCLUSION

We started by looking at how we understand the notion of challenge as it relates to young care leavers' involvement in social work education and we have explored how preconceptions of young people as 'challenging' and the challenges they themselves face impact upon the contribution they make to social work education. Our project started with engagement on a small scale at a grassroots level and has helped us in developing more holistic models of mental health within social work learning and teaching; setting mental health within a developmental context and particularly addressing the mental health needs of young people. However, we recognize, as Arnstein (1969) would argue, that real involvement demands the establishment of mechanisms within organizations which go beyond challenge and begin to genuinely redistribute power. This future development offers great opportunities for young people and the chance to enhance reciprocal relationships between academic organizations and service users involved in them. It also presents challenges to those organizations as to how they establish frameworks which enable service user involvement in management and support young service users whose voice is so important in social work, in these new roles. However, if social work education is to develop and grow, these issues will need to be addressed in future.

GOOD PRACTICE GUIDANCE FOR INVOLVING YOUNG CARE LEAVERS

- Young care leavers are a vulnerable and disempowered group of service users whose mental health needs are often not addressed in social work education.

- The involvement of young people in learning and teaching in social work education allows students to develop a more holistic perspective on mental health, seeing this aspect of human experience from a life-course focused, developmental perspective.

- Young care leavers bring their resilience and creativity to social work education but need reliable support from academics to do this.

- Young people emphasize the importance of presenting the whole person and not just the 'case' when developing materials for learning and teaching.

- When involving young service users in social work education, it is important to use empowering models of learning and teaching, such as problem-based learning.

The impact of young people's involvement on students can be profound and encourages students to critically reflect on their professional roles.

REFERENCES

Arnstein, S. (1969) 'A ladder of citizen participation.' *Journal of the American Institute of Planners 34*, 4, 216–224.

Banks, S. (2004) *Ethics, Accountability and the Social Professions*. Basingstoke: Palgrave MacMillan.

Barnett, S., Burrel, Y., Lupton, E., Green, L. and Wilks, T. (2005) 'Involving service users in the production of materials for social work education.' Presentation at Joint Social Work Education Conference, Loughborough, 16–19 July.

Basset, T., Campbell, P., Anderson, J. (2006) 'Service user/survivor involvement in mental health training and education: Overcoming the barriers.' *Social Work Education 25*, 4, 393–402.

Beresford, P. (2001) 'Service users, social policy and the future of welfare.' *Critical Social Policy 21*, 4, 494–512.

Braye, S. and Preston-Shoot, M. (2006) *Teaching, Learning and Assessment of Law in Social Work Education: A Resource Guide*. London: Social Care Institute for Excellence.

Broad, B. (2005) *Improving the Health and Well-being of Young People Leaving Care*. Lyme Regis: Random House Press.

Burgess, H. (1992) *Problem-led Learning for Social Work. The Enquiry and Action Learning Approach*. Bristol: University of Bristol.

Burgess, H. and Jackson, S. (1990) 'Enquiry and action learning: A new approach to social work education.' *Social Work Education 9*, 3, 3–19.

Croft, S. and Beresford, P. (1993) *Getting Involved: A Practical Manual*. London: Open Services Project and Joseph Rowntree Foundation.

Dance, C. and Rushton, A. (2005) 'Joining a new family. The views and experiences of young people placed with permanent families during middle childhood.' *Adoption and Fostering 29*, 1, 18–28.

Davies, J. and Wright, J. (2008) 'Children's voices: A review of the literature pertinent to looked-after children's views of mental health services.' *Child and Adolescent Mental Health 13*, 1, 26–31.

Department of Health (2000) *A Quality Strategy for Social Care*. London: Department of Health.

Department of Health (2002) *Listening, Learning and Responding. Department of Health Action Plan: Core Principles for the Involvement of Children and Young People*. London: The Stationery Office.

Department of Health (2004) *National Service Framework for Children, Young People and Maternity Services: Executive Summary*. London: The Stationery Office.

Dominelli, L. (2004) *Social Work Theory and Practice for a Changing Profession*. Oxford: Polity Press.

Erikson, E. (1971) *Identity: Youth and Crisis*. New York, NY: W.W. Norton.

Gilligan, R. (ed.) (2000) 'Promoting Resilience in Children in Foster Care.' In G. Kelly and R. Gilligan (eds) *Issues in Foster Care: Policy, Practice and Research*. London: Jessica Kingsley Publishers.

Green, L. and Wilks, T. (2009) 'Involving service users in a problem based model of teaching and learning.' *Social Work Education 28*, 2, 190–203.

Hart, R. (1992) *Children's Participation, from Tokenism to Citizenship*. Florence: UNICEF/ International Child Development Centre.

Hill, M., Davis, J., Prout, A. and Tisdall, K. (2004) 'Moving the participation agenda forward.' *Children and Society 18*, 2, 77–96.

HM Government (1989) *The Children Act 1989*. London: The Stationery Office.

Kelsey, B., Barnett, S., Green L. and Wilks, T. (2004) 'Young people on video: What young care leavers think about videos in social work education.' Presentation at Social Care Institute of Excellence Conference, Living and Learning Together, Birmingham University, July.

Levin, E. (2004) *Involving Service Users and Carers in Social Work Education*. Resource Guide No. 2. London: Bristol: Social Care Institute for Excellence.

Linhorst, D.M. (2002) 'A review of the use and potential of focus groups in social work research.' *Qualitative Social Work 1*, 2, 208–228.

Lockey, R., Sitzia, J., Gillingham, T., Millyard, T. *et al.* (2004) *Training for Service User Involvement in Health and Social Care Research: A Study of Training Provision and Participants' Experience.* Eastleigh: INVOLVE.

Manthorpe, J. (2000) 'Developing carers' contributions to social work training.' *Social Work Education 19*, 1, 19–27.

Marcia, J.E. (1966) 'Development and validation of ego-identity status.' *Journal of Personal and Social Psychology 3*, 5, 551–558.

Mental Health Foundation (2001) *Bright Futures: Promoting Children and Young People's Mental Health.* London: Mental Health Foundation.

Potter, R., Holmes, P. and Barton, H. (2002) 'Do we listen or do we assume? What teenagers want from a post abuse service.' *Psychiatric Bulletin 26*, 10, 377–379.

Prior, V., Lynch, M.A. and Glaser, D. (1999) 'Responding to child sexual abuse: An evaluation of social work by children and their carers.' *Child and Family Social Work 4*, 2, 131–143.

Quality Assurance Agency (QAA) (2000) *QAA Subject Benchmark Statement: Social Policy and Administration and Social Work.* Gloucester: QAA.

Quality Assurance Agency (QAA) (2008) *QAA Subject Benchmark Statement: Social Policy and Administration and Social Work.* Gloucester: QAA.

Read, J. and Reynolds, J. (eds) (1997) *Speaking Our Minds: An Anthology.* London: Macmillan.

Richardson, J. and Joughin, C. (2001) *The Mental Health Needs of Looked After Children.* London: Royal College of Psychiatrists.

Russell, M., Viner, M. and Taylor, B. (2005) 'Adult health and social outcomes for children who have been in public care: Population based study.' *Pediatrics 115*, 4, 894–899.

Sanders, J. and Munford, R. (2007) 'Speaking from the margins: Implications for education and practice of young women's experience of marginalisation.' *Social Work Education 26*, 2, 185–199.

Stein, M. (2005) *Resilience and Young People Leaving Care. Overcoming the Odds.* York: Joseph Rowntree Foundation.

United Nations (1989) *United Nations Convention on the Rights of the Child.* Available at www.everychildmatters.gov.uk/_files/589DD6D3A29C929ACB148DB3F13B 01E7.pdf, accessed on 12 May 2009.

CHAPTER 13

Conclusion: The Way Forward for Service User Involvement and Recovery

Jenny Weinstein

INTRODUCTION

Service users writing or commenting on different subjects in this book reiterate the same themes, albeit in different contexts; they want to see a Recovery approach being adopted by all mental health services and this means being involved in all aspects of the design, delivery, evaluation and commissioning of those services. The Recovery approach is now an official strategy promoted by the government (Department of Health 2001) but, at the time of writing, service user contributors to this book are describing a very variable experience in practice that seems to depend to a large extent on the attitudes of individual practitioners (see Chapter 7). In this concluding chapter, we will summarize the book's themes and, in so doing, critique some of the initiatives that have been introduced or proposed to overcome the apparent barriers to progress towards Recovery – in particular,

- challenging the medical model

- enabling service users to have more involvement in their own treatment and care

- tackling stigma and social exclusion

- strengthening the service user movement.

CHALLENGING THE MEDICAL MODEL

Reflecting retrospectively on her mental health breakdown in Chapter 5, Aloyse Raptopoulos describes a range of acute symptoms that she suffered and wonders how the psychiatrist decided on a diagnosis of depression when her symptoms could have been associated with a number of identified mental illnesses. Humphrey Greaves in Chapter 3 talks about how humiliating and degrading it was for him to receive a diagnosis (label). Smith (2009) relates his experience of starting to hear voices, being diagnosed with paranoid schizophrenia, being sectioned and being given heavy doses of medication. He did not Recover until he encountered a member of the Hearing Voices Network (a charity linking local self-help groups established in 1989: see www.hearing-voices.org/information. htm) who advised him to challenge the voices and refuse to do what they said if he did not want to. This advice led Smith to realize that the voices were part of him and therefore not so frightening. He taught himself to control them without medication and concludes: 'Facing them and working with them has changed my life and made me feel optimistic' (Smith 2009, p.10).

Challenges to the medical model such as these are reinforced by Bentall, a renowned psychiatrist and researcher (Bentall and HG Publishing 2003), who argues that it is not possible to divide madness into a small number of diagnosable diseases such as schizophrenia or manic depression. Bentall goes on to point out that for a categorical system of diagnosis to work, patients must all fit the criteria for a particular disease, which as Raptopoulos points out, does not happen in real life. Bentall (Bentall and HG Publishing 2003) concludes that the reason for the very similar symptoms that are observed in what we know as schizophrenia, depression and mania indicate that they are not really distinct and separate disorders. He supports what user authors of this book argue, that mental health professionals and service users need to share information and explore together the best approach to Recovery because 'you can't consider the brain in isolation from the social world and the experiences people have' (Bentall and HG Publishing 2003, p.1).

The mental illness labels challenged by Bentall, and by many in the service user movement, serve only to feed into stigma and discrimination and deepen an unreal division between those who are 'mentally ill' and those who are 'sane'. While acknowledging the efficacy of medical treatments to reduce certain distressing symptoms and recognizing that some people find a diagnosis helpful to explain their symptoms, it is argued here that labels such as 'schizophrenic', 'bipolar' and 'paranoid' need to be used with considerable caution and with an awareness that, as more is learnt about mental illness, it may become possible to dispense with these terms altogether.

ENABLING SERVICE USERS TO HAVE MORE INVOLVEMENT IN THEIR OWN TREATMENT AND CARE

Care planning

Service user authors in this book constantly reiterate their demands to be fully involved in their own treatment and care. Although it is a key principle of the Care Planning Approach (CPA) framework (Department of Health 2006) that service users should be involved, in 2007 a patient survey (Health Care Commission 2007) found that only 50 per cent of service users understood their care plan. This appears to be an ongoing problem (Hounsell and Owens 2005; Warner 2005) that clearly requires a revised approach.

A new tool called Wellness Recovery Action Plans (WRAPs) (Copeland 2002) may assist improved involvement in care planning. WRAPs were not mentioned by any of our service user authors, possibly because they have only recently been introduced to the UK from the USA. WRAPS are a form of user-focused care planning aimed to maximize empowerment and choice for the individual whether they are ill, in crisis, in Recovery or well. It is suggested that if they were introduced in a comprehensive way across all service users and services, they could transform the user-professional relationship in the way proposed by the personalization agenda.

Advocacy

Although all service users have their own views about what they want and need, some are less confident about expressing themselves and require support. For example, service users have said that they need advocates to support them in negotiating Independent Budgets (IBs: see Chapter 7). The government has expressed its commitment to advocacy:

> Advocacy is a way of making sure that the voices of those people most in need are heard, thereby enabling everyone to access the services and support to which they are entitled. It means taking action to help people say what they want, to secure their rights, to represent their interests and obtain the services that best meet their needs. If people can't do that, in this area in particular, it can have an impact on recovery. (Winerton 2006)

For these reasons, the Government places a high value on advocacy as a way of helping vulnerable people to get the most out of services and of maximising their independence and autonomy. But at the same time Advocacy can also help the professionals provide a better service. Advocates, for instance, can help doctors and nurses and other health and social care professionals understand service users wishes by:

- helping them prepare for consultations and care planning meetings

- helping them to feel able to say what they want.

It is interesting that none of the service users who contributed to the book mentioned having had access to advocacy and Julie Gosling in Chapter 2 describes how hard her organization has had to fight to provide genuinely independent advocacy to people and that this is often unpaid. Resources are a major problem. Since April 2009, statutory access to an Independent Mental Health Advocate (IMHA) has been available under the Mental Health Act 2007 to patients subject to compulsory detention or those who are subject to the Mental Capacity Act 2005. The automatic right to advocacy is thus restricted to these statutory requirements. Access for other service users is patchy, and depends on the investment in advocacy services by different statutory bodies. This can result in a postcode lottery for service users so that accessible independent advocacy is unlikely to be consistantly available unless users establish their own peer advocacy groups.

Individual Budgets (IBs)

The government aims to mainstream individual budgets by 2011 and to have achieved a 30 per cent take-up of IBs by 2011/12. Although self-directed and tailored support should be available to aid Recovery, a number of reasons have been identified for the relatively low take-up. Local authorities have been somewhat daunted by the complexity of making such a radical change and have responded by creating bureaucratic barriers to take-up, while many service users have expressed reluctance to adopt IBs due to the real or perceived burdens of financial and/or personnel management that they bring (Samuel 2008). A further concern is that, with the introduction of IBs, the funding for mental health day care centres, which can provide a hub and a secure sanctuary, may be threatened (National Social Inclusion Programme, NIMHE and CSIP 2006).

Implementing the targets for take-up of IBs will require a deep and significant shift in the relationship between professionals and service users as social workers change their roles from care managers to navigators and sign posters. There is no prescribed format about how this will work and the interface between health and social care will need to be resolved. For example, one mental health service user complained that he could use his IB to pay for tickets to football matches but not to purchase the therapy he wanted to improve his mental health. This is because his personal budget related only to *social* care while therapy was seen as something to be paid for by *health*. In an ideal world a holistic approach would be achieved by pooling social services IBs with the personal health budgets proposed by the Darzi review for people with long-term conditions, including mental illness (Darzi 2008; Department of Health 2009). The personal health budgets are due to be piloted in 2009 and are controversial within the NHS. For example, McIntosh (2009) reports that the King's Fund has questioned whether the new system may increase inequalities and managers have concerns about the complexity of commissioning a multiplicity of individual person-centred services. On the other hand, the mental health charity MIND supports the proposals, seeing them as empowering service users to choose their own treatments and improving doctor–patient relationships.

Talking therapies

One particular demand of service users has been for talking therapies. The Improving Access to Psychological Therapies (IAPT) programme (Department of Health and Care Services Improvement Partnership 2006) seeks to provide improved access to psychological therapies for people who require the help of mental health services. It also responds to service users' requests for more personalized services based around their individual needs. In debates about the issues at a psychological therapies conference (Browne 2008), delegates acknowledged that many people prefer alternative psychodynamically orientated therapies which may not be permitted as part of the programme because they are not deemed to be evidence based. Doubts were also expressed about the degree of genuine choice (for example, about race or gender of the therapist) that service users would have. In response to concerns, a Statement of Intent launched by the government (Johnson 2008) pledged to tackle the stigma that often stops people with mental health problems from accessing psychological therapies and to ensure that people will be offered a choice of evidence-based therapies to meet their needs rather than being strictly confined to the short-term cognitive behavioural models.

TACKLING STIGMA AND SOCIAL EXCLUSION

Anti-stigma campaign

The Anti-Stigma Campaign in England (Time to Change 2009) has taken off with newspaper and TV advertisements featuring high profile celebrities such as Stephen Fry, the distinguished writer and actor, and Alastair Campbell, press aide to former Prime Minister, Tony Blair, who speak frankly about their own experiences of mental ill health. In addition local and national activities have been sponsored, such as community projects to promote well-being and social inclusion, national events to encourage and promote exercise as a vital ingredient to improve mental health, and education projects to raise awareness among those who have an impact on people with mental health issues. Through the Open Up network, a specific user-led initiative to challenge prejudice and discrimination, members can access support, advice, training and inspiration for their work challenging mental health discrimination. Inevitably, campaigns such as Time to Change have a challenging task in influencing public perceptions of mental illness in the face of, arguably, the much higher media profile given to the relatively small number of tragic incidents (see, for example, Siddique 2009) when things have gone wrong because someone with serious mental health difficulties has not been provided with the support they need.

Social Inclusion

The government's programme for challenging social exclusion in mental health was launched in 2004 (Office of the Deputy Prime Minister 2004). A new framework for monitoring outcomes was announced five years later (National Social Inclusion Programme 2009), which suggests that outcomes should be monitored only where campaigns have 'succeeded' to ensure that people do not feel they are being set up to fail. It is suggested here that the very use of the word 'succeed' continues to imply a culture whereby the expectations of service users are being set by others rather than by themselves.

The proposed outcomes are that more people will:

- volunteer in mainstream settings (it would be interesting to know whether 'mainstream' settings means settings that are not mental health orientated. If so, this entirely misses the point when there is so much evidence, not least in this book, that mental health experts by experience can make such excellent interventions in mental health settings through their volunteering.)

- participate in community activities

- make and retain more friends and social contacts

- prepare for employment

- enter paid employment

- access education and training

- improve their physical health

- take regular exercise

- improve their quality of life and self-esteem

- live in independent accommodation

- receive appropriate benefits and financial advice

- receive direct payments or individual budgets

- express satisfaction with the service

- be more involved in planning and delivery of services.

While some of these outcomes may be very positive for some individuals, what of the person who wants to be a loner and write poetry or make music? What about the person who wants to spend more time parenting their children? What about the person who does not want to manage direct payments or an individual budget? What about the person who feels too unwell to work? All of these individuals can still 'succeed' in Recovery terms if they identify and meet their *own* aspirations. This can particularly be the case for service users from different cultures whose own perspectives may not fit in with Eurocentric criteria. For example, an approach developed in New Zealand illustrates the importance of valuing a person's cultural origins based on an understanding of Recovery being about people regaining a sense of their own identity so that they can reintegrate into their own communities in their own way (Lapsley, Waimarie and Black 2002).

A slightly more person-centred model, but a predetermined system nevertheless is the Recovery Star approach (Mental Health Providers'

Forum 2009) that was developed bottom up in partnership with service users (see Figure 13.1). In this model the person is put at the centre of the star with their points of recovery again covering predetermined aspects rather than leaving service users to set their own goals.

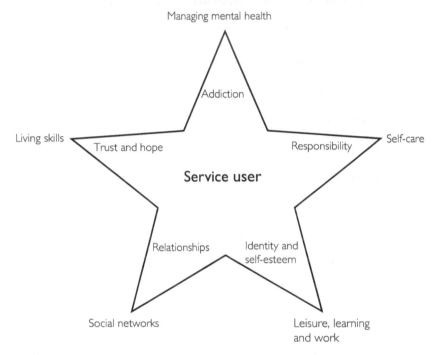

Figure 13.1: Recovery star

Rather than measuring the achievements of service users, a model known as DREEM (Developing Recovery-Enhancing Environments Measure: Allott, Clark and Slade 2006; Ridgway and Press 2004) has been developed by service users to measure the degree to which mental health services are geared to promoting Recovery.

Employment

Finding a job and making a contribution are, nevertheless, important aspirations for some service users, as described by Humphrey Greaves (Chapter 3) and Aloyse Raptopoulos (Chapter 6). The Welfare Reform Act 2009 aims to encourage more people with disabilities to return to work by making much closer links between entitlement to benefits and jobseeking. Extra support has been promised to people with mental and physical disabilities in terms of job preparation and job finding which would be compulsory, following assessment, for those on benefit who are deemed to be employable. However, the mental health think-tank, the Sainsbury Centre for Mental Health, is concerned about the risk of 'requiring people to undertake activities that are not proven to help them to get jobs simply to maintain their benefits' (Greatley 2009, p.35). So, to combat this possibility, MIND (2009) is campaigning for:

- employment advisers with skills and training in mental health

- an explicit safeguard for those who are unable to comply with requirements due to mental health problems

- welfare reform proposals to be complemented by government strategies for improving workplace mental health

- increased expectations on employers to create improved opportunities for jobseekers with mental health problems.

And we cannot ignore the impact of the broader worldwide economic crisis where even those with long experience and expertise in the world of work are facing rising levels of unemployment.

A holistic approach

While employment is clearly vital, some service user authors in this book explained that their illness can make holding down a job too stressful. Nevertheless, they are still keen to undertake meaningful activities such as volunteering, creative arts, culture, sports and education, all of which can offer a way back from exclusion into the community and towards Recovery. In Chapter 8, service users describe the positive impact on their own mental health that being involved in raising mental health awareness has had and in Chapters 10, 11 and 12, the valuable contributions that users can make to research and training are evidenced with the additional spin-off in relation to participants' improved confidence and self-esteem.

STRENGTHENING THE SERVICE USER MOVEMENT

For many years there were calls to establish a National User Involvement Network (NUIN). Such a body was launched with high hopes in 2007 and an aim to support local user groups but, like many umbrella and national groups, NUIN appears to be struggling to find its way and its role, possibly because service user involvement is often a specifically service or project-focused activity.

To provide a more locally based model, the government gave a commitment that:

> By 2010, each locality (defined as that area covered by a Council with social services responsibilities) should have a user-led organization, modelled on existing CILs (Centres for Independent Living). (Department of Health 2005, p.91)

The small number of effective CILs work towards independent living by providing people with support to make choices and have control such as:

- support to help people to self-assess their needs

- support to use direct payments

- advocacy and support for self-advocacy

- peer support

- advice and information.

CILs also offer services to meet people's needs, such as assistance in recruiting and employing personal assistants, employment support projects, supported housing services and peer support services (Morris 2007, p.6).

When organizations were consulted about what form an overarching user-led organization should take (Morris 2007), there was a general view expressed that one organization could not undertake all the tasks and represent all the groups envisaged in the *Improving the Life Chances* pledge (Department of Health 2005; Prime Minister's Strategy Unit 2005). It was therefore suggested that there could be a network or federation of a range of different organizations which might offer a concrete or a virtual 'hub'.

Although the government made the pledge to establish CILs and user-led organizations in 2005 and gave grants for their development, CILs have still not taken off in many areas. No service user consulted as part of this book even mentioned this model as a key requirement. One barrier suggested by Morris (2007) may be that the different groups of people who need support in their daily lives use different terms to describe themselves and what they want even though they may be in agreement with each other that the most important thing is to have choice and control over the support needed. It is suggested here that there may be some contradictions between introducing personalization, so that people can live their own independent lives integrated within the community while at the same time legislating from above for user-led organizations.

CONCLUSION AND GOOD PRACTICE GUIDANCE

A number of key themes have been identified for taking user involvement and Recovery forward (Care Services Improvement Partnership, Royal College of Psychiatrists and Social Care Institute for Excellence 2007), many of which are reflected in the views expressed by authors in this book. These have been conflated, adapted and summarized below.

- Recovery is about focusing on people's strengths and their identity as a *person* rather than on their symptoms and their identity as a *patient*.

- Optimism is central to Recovery. At their lowest ebb, people need to have their potential and their skills recognized and valued. Humphrey Greaves illustrates so clearly in Chapter 3 how important it is to encounter people who trusted and believed in him after years of having been dismissed. Phrases like 'You'll never...' are anathema to Recovery approaches.

- Recovery, as Julie Gosling says in Chapter 2, is about getting back in the driving seat and steering your own life. Without adequate information, choice and encouragement, this can be hard for someone suffering from a debilitating illness.

- An individual's own personal cultural background, sexuality, belief system or spirituality can provide significant strength and direction for their Recovery, especially if this is recognized and respected by professionals who work with them.

- As summed up succinctly by a service user who wishes to remain anonymous, everyone needs 'someone to love, something to do and somewhere to live'. If relationships, activities and housing are adequately addressed, this will go a long way towards supporting Recovery.

- Recovery requires acceptance by the family, the community and mainstream services, which means not being excluded, discriminated against or stereotyped.

- Language is critical; labelling is counterproductive for Recovery.

- Treatment is much more likely to be effective if it is agreed in partnership and if evidence for intervention is made explicit and fully explained.

- Recovery approaches require creative imaginative approaches that go beyond current bureaucratic risk-averse and formulaic interventions and this can be progressed with the help of effective user-led research.

- Mental health staff at all levels play a critical role in Recovery. Whether from a consultant psychiatrist or a support worker, what service users say they value most is people who treat them with the compassion required by an individual who is unwell and may be vulnerable; people who actively listen to them; people who respect them for who they are; and people who believe they have a future. In other words, mental health professionals who can show 'humility, humanity and hope' (Secker 2009).

The strength and resilience of mental health service users can be evidenced by the significant gains they have made over four decades of campaigning as chronicled in this book. Some user authors remain understandably cynical, given the perceived slow pace of change; others are optimistic that through their continued involvement in service development, campaigning and training, they will eventually see the rhetoric of social inclusion, involvement and Recovery translated into their day-to-day experience of mental health services.

THE LAST WORD COMES FROM A SERVICE USER, HUMPHREY GREAVES

In this book, we have shown some of the numerous examples of mental health service user involvement and how it is occurring today. As a service user myself, I, Humphrey Greaves, would like you to imagine that you are a member of our Hope circle in which each of us says what we hope for. First, it is my turn and I hope for:

- All service users to be listened to, respected, and valued.

- All service users to be seen as a positive influence on both their own health and that of others, instead of being seen as a problem or a nasty stain on the statistics printout, or just as a burden on society.

- Recognition that we have a valuable input to make: if only some-one would listen instead of giving the answer before the question has been asked.

- Service users to receive care when we ask for it, not have it given when we are all but at death's door, as we are so often turned away from medical services where early intervention might have prevented a protracted illness.

If Winston Churchill had not been listened to, respected and valued during World War II, many of us would not be alive today. Winston Churchill suffered from mental illness. Who have you not listened to?

Now it is your turn to hope…

REFERENCES

Allott, P., Clark, M. and Slade, M. (2006) *Taking DREEM Forward: Background and Summary of Experience with REE/DREEM So Far and Recommendations.* Report pre-pared for Director of Mental Health Research, Department of Health, London. Available from authors at mentalhealthrecovery@blueyonder.co.uk

Bentall, R. and HG Publishing (2003) *A New Look at Psychosis.* Chalvington: Human Givens Institute. Available at www.hgi.org.uk/archive/newlook-psychosis3.htm, accessed on 12 May 2009.

Browne, S. (2008) 'Psychological therapies in the NHS.' *Therapy Today,* December, 4–6.

Care Services Improvement Partnership, Royal College of Psychiatrists and Social Care Institute for Excellence (2007) *A Common Purpose: Recovery in Future Mental Health Services.* London: SCIE.

Copeland, M.E. (2002) *Wellness Recovery Action Plan.* West Dummerston, VT: Peach Press.

Darzi, Lord (2008) *High Quality Care for All: NHS Next Stage Review Final Report,* Cm 7432. London: The Stationery Office.

Department of Health (2001) *The Journey to Recovery: The Government's Vision for Mental Health Care.* London: The Stationery Office.

Department of Health (2005) *Improving the Life Chances of Disabled People.* London: Department of Health.

Department of Health (2006) *Community Care Assessments and Plans.* London: The Stationery Office.

Department of Health (2009) *Health Bill 2009.* London: Department of Health. Available at www.dh.gov.uk/en/Publicationsandstatistics/Legislation/Actsand bills/DH_093280, accessed on 12 May 2009.

Department of Health and Care Services Improvement Partnership (2006) *Improving Access to Psychological Therapies.* London: Department of Health. Available at www.dh.gov.uk/en/Publicationsandstatistics/Publications/Publications PolicyAndGuidance/DH_073470, accessed on 12 May 2009.

Greatley, A. (2009) 'Workfare protests face New Labour.' Letters. *Guardian,* 25 February. Available at www.guardian.co.uk/politics/2009/feb/25/welfare-re-form-bill-uk, accessed on 12 May 2009.

Health Care Commission (2007) *Community Mental Health Survey 2007.* London: National Centre for Social Research.

HM Government (2005) *Mental Capacity Act 2005.* London: The Stationery Office.

HM Government (2007) *Mental Health Act 2007.* London: The Stationery Office.

HM Government (2009) *Welfare Reform Act 2009.* London: The Stationery Office.

Hounsell, J. and Owens, C. (2005) 'User research in control.' *Mental Health Today,* May, 29–33.

Johnson, A. (2008) 'Statement of Intent November 2008.' Speech by Alan Johnson, Secretary of State for Health, at the New Savoy Partnership Conference, London, November. Available at www.iapt.nhs.uk/2008/12/statement-of-in-tent-november-2008, accessed on 12 May 2009.

Lapsley, H., Waimarie, L.N. and Black, R. (2002) *'Kia Mauri Tau!': Narratives of Recovery from Disabling Mental Health Problems.* Wellington: Mental Health Commission.

McIntosh, K. (2009) 'Personal health budgets: The patient is always right.' *Health Service Journal,* 2 March. Available at www.hsj.co.uk/personal-health-budgets-the-patient-is-always-right/1988779.article, accessed on 12 May 2009.

Mental Health Providers Forum (2009) *The Recovery Star Approach.* London: Mental Health Providers Forum. Available at www.mhpf.org.uk/recoveryStarAp-proach.asp, accessed on 12 May 2009.

MIND (2009) *Welfare Reform Bill 2009: Campaigns Briefing.* London: MIND. Available at www.mind.org.uk/NR/rdonlyres/7D90CD56-EC3E-47F2-B820-247F38 573261/7400/BriefingonWelfareReformBill2009forcampaigners.pdf, accessed on 12 May 2009.

Morris, J. (2007) *Centres for Independent Living/Local User-Led Organizations: A Discussion Paper.* London: Department of Health.

National Social Inclusion Programme, National Institute for Mental Health in England and Care Services Improvement Partnership (2006) *From Segregation to Inclusion: Commissioning Guidance on Day Services for People with Mental Health Problems.* London: Department of Health. Available at www.dh.gov.uk/en/ Publicationsandstatistics/Publications/PublicationsPolicyAndGuidance/ DH_4131061, accessed on 12 May 2009.

National Social Inclusion Programme (2009) *Outcomes Framework for Mental Health Services*. London: National Institute for Mental Health in England. Available at www.socialinclusion.org.uk/publications/Broadened_Social_Inclusion_Outcomes_Framework.pdf, accessed on 12 May 2009.

Office of the Deputy Prime Minister (ODPM) (2004) *Mental Health and Social Exclusion: Social Exclusion Unit Report*. London: ODPM.

Prime Minister's Strategy Unit (2005) *Improving the Life Chances of Disabled People: Final Report*. London: Cabinet Office. Available at www.cabinetoffice.gov.uk/media/cabinetoffice/strategy/assets/disability.pdf, accessed on 12 May 2009.

Ridgway, P.A. and Press, A. (2004) *Assessing the Recovery Commitment of Your Mental Health Services: A User's Guide to the Developing Recovery Enhancing Environments Measure (DREEM)*. UK pilot version. Recovery Devon (Partnerships in Mental Health). Available at www.recoverydevon.co.uk/html/downloads/DREEM%20total%20dft4%20no%20tc.pdf, accessed on 12 May 2009.

Samuel, M. (2008) *Direct Payments, Personal Budgets and Individual Budgets*. Community Care Expert Guides. Available at www.communitycare.co.uk/Articles/2008/08/24/102669/direct-payments-personal-budgets-and-individual-budgets.html, accessed on 12 May 2009.

Secker, J. (2009) Personal communication, at workshop on User Involvement in HE, Anglia Ruskin University, 18 February.

Siddique, H. (2009) 'Man jailed for life for stabbing policemen to death.' *Guardian*, 25 March. Available at www.guardian.co.uk/uk/2009/mar/25/ukcrime-mental-health, accessed on 12 May 2009.

Smith, D. (2009) 'I talk back to the voices in my head.' *Guardian*, 4 April. Available at www.guardian.co.uk/lifeandstyle/2009/apr/04/mental-health-health-and-wellbeing, accessed on 12 May 2009.

Time to Change (2009) *What We're Doing*. London: Time to Change. Available at www.time-to-change.org.uk/what-were-doing, accessed on 12 May 2009.

Warner, L. (2005) 'Review of the literature on the Care Programme Approach.' In Sainsbury Centre for Mental Health (ed.) *Back on Track?* London: Sainsbury Centre for Mental Health. Available at www.scmh.org.uk/publications/back_on_track.aspx?ID=436, accessed on 12 May 2009.

Winterton, R. (2006) Speech by Rosie Winterton, Minister of State for Health: Sainsbury Centre Conference, Mental Health Advocacy: Facing the Future, London, 28 March. Available at www.dh.gov.uk/en/News/Speeches/Speecheslist/DH_4134600, accessed on 12 May 2009.

The Contributors

Julie Gosling is a disabled woman, and survivor of domestic violence and homelessness who founded Advocacy in Action in the early 1990s. Since then, Julie has supported the empowerment of service users both nationally and internationally. She is extensively involved in professional education and contributes as a service user regulator for social work education.

Humphrey Greaves has been a user of mental health services since 1981 but has continued to work despite his illness. Through his experience, he has been able to help other service users and is currently a BME User Development Worker with Southwark MIND and a self-employed Personal Coach and NLP Practitioner.

Liz Green coordinates the Masters in Social Work at Goldsmiths College, University of London. She worked as a social worker for 16 years with children and people with mental health issues before teaching at Bromley College and then Goldsmiths. She has published widely on her work involving young care leavers in social work education.

Jewish Care Education Project provides a ground-breaking service to raise awareness and acceptance of those with mental health needs. Members deliver creative presentations that bring mental health issues to life and deal with them in straight-talking, easily understandable language. By educating people they break down prejudice, fight ignorance and promote inclusion.

Dr Philip Kemp is Principal Lecturer at London South Bank University. He is a mental health nurse with an extensive background of working with people who have experienced enduring mental health difficulties within health and social care settings. Currently, he is researching and developing service user involvement in professional education.

Professor Tony Leiba is Emeritus Professor of Mental Health at London South Bank University. He supervises MPhil and PhD students and researches mental health, interprofessional education and practice, evidence-based practice and conflict management.

Aloyse Raptopoulos is a musician, singer and writer of African-French-Greek descent who lived in North and South America before moving in 2000 to London, where she experienced a breakdown. A former service user, she is now an independent trainer and consultant in mental health, and a part-time lecturer at London South Bank University.

Southwark MIND is a user-led local MIND Association engaged in campaigning for better services for mental health users and facilitating peer support groups. Members of Southwark MIND participate in decision-making bodies about mental health for both their local Mental Health Trust and for the local council's mental health services.

Jenny Weinstein is an independent consultant in health and social care. Her experience spans management and development in the statutory, voluntary and education sectors; she was previously Principal Lecturer in Mental Health at London South Bank University. Her research and publication activities focus on interprofessional collaboration, diversity and service user involvement.

Tom Wilks is Senior Lecturer in Social Work at London South Bank University. He was a social worker and manager in mental health services before moving into teaching. He collaborated with Liz Green to publish and promote their involvement of young service users in developing teaching materials for social work education.

Subject Index

218

Author Index